THE BACKGROUND TO ANTHROPOSOPHICAL THERAPEUTIC SPEECH

THE BACKGROUND TO ANTHROPOSOPHICAL THERAPEUTIC SPEECH

Edited by Dietrich von Bonin

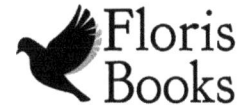

Translated from German by David Macgregor

First published in 2008 by Verlag Förderstiftung Anthroposophischer Medizin as *Materialien zur Therapeutischen Sprachgestaltung*

This English edition published in 2012 by Floris Books. Second printing 2024

Publication of this translation has been made possible through the generous help of the Anthroposophical Medical Trust, the Anthroposophical Society in Great Britain, Hermes Trust, Michael Wilson Trust, the Therapeutic Speech Association, and others.

© 2008 Medical Section at the Goetheanum, Dornach, Switzerland
Translation © 2012 Floris Books

All rights reserved. No part of this publication may be reproduced without the prior permission of Floris Books, Edinburgh
www.florisbooks.co.uk

British Library CIP Data available
ISBN 978-086315-876-6

Contents

Foreword by Michael Glöckler — 9

Introduction by Dietrich von Bonin — 11

1 Pioneers of Anthroposophical Therapeutic Speech

Martha Hemsoth by Dietrich von Bonin — 17
    Speech exercises by Martha Hemsoth — 30
    The mystery of effective speech by Martha Hemsoth — 33

Hildegard Jordi A brief autobiography — 37
    Therapeutic methods for psychiatric illnesses by Hilde Jordi — 41

Dora Gutbrod (Autobiography) — 73

2 Therapeutic Speech and Rudolf Steiner

A Therapeutic Exercise: An Angegebenes sieh innig hin — 89

A Second Therapeutic Exercise: Richtig recht rechnen — 99

A Third Therapeutic Exercise: Ich atme Kraft des Lebens — 105

Reminiscences of Rudolf Steiner by Willi Kux — 109

Esoteric Lesson by Rudolf Steiner — 115

3 Aspects of Speech Formation

Upright Walking, Speech Movement, Eurythmy
   by Gisbert Husemann   123

The Fourfold and Fivefold Nature of the Human Being
   by Dietrich von Bonin   139

Some Experiences with Speech Formation by Ida Rüchardt   151

Speech Formation in the Waldorf School by Ilse Schuckmann   175

4 Reports on the Development of Therapeutic Speech since 1976

Report on the Further Training Course for Speech Formation
   Practitioners by Caroline Wispler   183

The Origins and New Beginning of Therapeutic Speech
   by Ursula Ostermai   193

Notes   199

Bibliography   202

Index   204

Translator's Note on Pronunciation

The vowel sounds in the text follow German pronunciation. Equivalent English approximations are as follows:

    A — as in 'ah' (bath)
    E — as in 'eh' (bait)
    I — as in 'ee' (beet)
    O — as in 'oh' (boat)
    U — as in 'oo' (boot)
    Au — as in 'ow' (bout)
    Ei — as in the personal pronoun 'I' (bite)

    Ch — as in Scots 'loch,' not as in 'cheese'

Foreword

Anthroposophic therapeutic speech is more than an integral component of anthroposophic medicine's specialist field of the therapeutic arts. It also helps in training physicians to develop a differentiated understanding of the organization of the I as the spiritual regulator of the organism's warmth processes and their healing power.

Through the intentionality in a consciously formed process of speaking, the warmth organism is activated from within the I. As a consequence, through the breath which is thereby changed and its effect on the life of the body, the clients intervene in their whole constitution and regulate it. The beginnings of this new concept of therapy go back to a few pioneers whose work until now — with a few exceptions — lived on only as oral tradition.

Dietrich von Bonin, with his colleagues, researchers and collaborators, has brought together in this publication a large part of this invaluable background material. In the name of the co-workers of the Medical Section at the Goetheanum I would like to thank them most warmly for this.

I should like to recommend this book not only to physicians, speech and language therapists, and to anthroposophical therapeutic speech practitioners, but also to speech artists, actors, teachers and educators, as well as all who love speech in its many forms of expression.

Anyone who enjoys eyewitness accounts of Rudolf Steiner and his work, and of rehearsals with Marie Steiner, the inaugurator of speech formation, will welcome this book.

Michaela Glöckler
Medical Section at the Goetheanum

Introduction

Therapeutic speech as a specialist field in the anthroposophical therapeutic arts is spreading and becoming more recognized. Questions frequently arise as to how it may be defined and how its quality may be preserved. This has led to a need to reflect on the origins of this therapy which had its beginnings in the first decades of the twentieth century.

As with many pioneers, the first practitioners of therapeutic speech were enthusiastically devoted to the new possibilities of this work, and written accounts were only made at a relatively late stage. In 1978 Christa Slezak-Schindler published her book on artistic speaking for children of school age, followed later by books on other themes concerning therapy through speech formation, which she called artistic speech therapy. Two further books on the healing power of speech, by Agathe Lorenz-Poschmann, appeared in 1983. Then a series of large annual conferences for all the different anthroposophical artistic therapies took place between 1989 and 1998 on the initiative of Dr Michaela Glöckler. Four basic volumes on anthroposophic artistic therapy sprang from these conferences, including one on therapeutic speech.[1] However the scanty material on its beginnings had hardly been uncovered and was largely unknown.

The present work aims to fill that gap by making available reports, articles and other material on the origin and development of our profession. The first part has biographies of three colleagues, two of whom are almost unknown even within the profession: Martha Hemsoth and Hilde Jordi, who dedicated themselves with great devotion to a task which at first did not appear to suit them.

We have Emanuel Zeylmans van Emmichoven to thank for drawing attention to the existence of Martha Hemsoth. Inquiries led to the Ita Wegman Archive, which made available what was preserved of the correspondence between Martha Hemsoth and Ita Wegman.

I became aware of Hilde Jordi's life through an apparent coincidence when I was requested to recite some texts at her funeral. And so this remarkably dedicated colleague's valuable account of how she developed completely new approaches to therapy in psychiatry found its way into this collection.

The destinies of both women have in common that crises took them away from their vocation for the artistic into a medical and therapeutic direction. We are reminded here of the expression attributed to Ita Wegman, 'the sacrificed art'. Something else in common, which may appear surprising, is that both were asked to play the Guardian of the Threshold in Rudolf Steiner's mystery drama and that neither actually did so. Their destinies were both also quite hard toward the end of their lives. Ita Wegman's colleague died young as the result of an accident while Hilde Jordi (who worked in central Switzerland) spent the evening of her life very much in need of care, which was provided through the devoted companionship of her life-long friend, Helene Pflugshaupt. Motifs in the destinies of both recall one of Marie Steiner's remarks, passed on by Kurt Hendewerk, 'In eurythmy you place yourself into a higher order; in speech formation you work with the dangerous forces of your previous incarnations.'[2] Are the origins of their illnesses perhaps concealed within these forces?

Dora Gutbrod was one of Marie Steiner's closest pupils, worked for 23 years under her direction and on the Goetheanum stage for a total of 50 years. Based on this experience, she wanted to make the forces effective in speech formation more widely accessible, and put all her efforts into the development of therapeutic speech formation. Through her close friendship with the then director of the Ita Wegman Clinic, Madeleine van Deventer, and under her aegis, she began treating cases — including depression, hearing loss and exhaustion — through therapeutic speech. Marie Steiner's work with Dora Gutbrod over the decades was a service to the word and to speech extending far beyond the art of acting; for the pioneers mentioned in this book it formed the foundation for taking the step from art to therapy.

Part 2 contains the sources of three specific therapeutic speech exercises by Rudolf Steiner which were difficult to document, as either they had not been published before or publication was difficult to trace. The exercises appear with all their indications and in the form in which they first appeared in print. They each have an up-to-date commentary from a current perspective.

An entire esoteric lesson, which describes the effects of different breathing processes, has been included in connection with one of the exercises in order to shed more light on it.

Part 3 has a collection of articles on various aspects of therapeutic speech work. One is by Gisbert Husemann on upright movement, speech movement and eurythmy. It underlines the inner affinity of speech formation to eurythmy and is a remarkable example of succinct Goethean

description. Then there is a fundamental study of how the five lower aspects of the human being are revealed in speech. Ida Rüchardt reflects on Rudolf Steiner's speech exercises, and adds many examples of her own, to help prepare and deepen artistic speaking.

This chapter concludes with reflections of a longstanding speech formation teacher at the Hanover Waldorf school, Ilse Schuckmann, on the many tasks and challenges, but also the attraction of such a challenging profession.

Part 4 has reports about the development of therapeutic speech between 1976 and the present day. Of these, the report by Caroline Wispler on the large conference of 1976 appears not merely as a review but also as a suggested pattern for the future. As a result of that conference, Dora Gutbrod founded a training in Dornach which was directed for many years by her pupil, Ursula Ostermai. Her thoughts on the past and ideas for the future round off the chapter.

I would like particularly to thank my fellow authors Barbara Denjean-von Stryk, Ursula Ostermai, Ralf Unterbusch and Ilse Schuckmann for their contributions and collegial collaboration, and Ruth Andrea and Dorit Dirlam for tracking down texts and their numerous helpful commentaries. Peter Selg and Gunhild Pörksen of the Ita Wegman Archive kindly gave permission to print quotations from letters, as did Walter Kugler of the Executors of Rudolf Steiner's Estate.

Dietrich von Bonin

1

Pioneers of Anthroposophical Therapeutic Speech

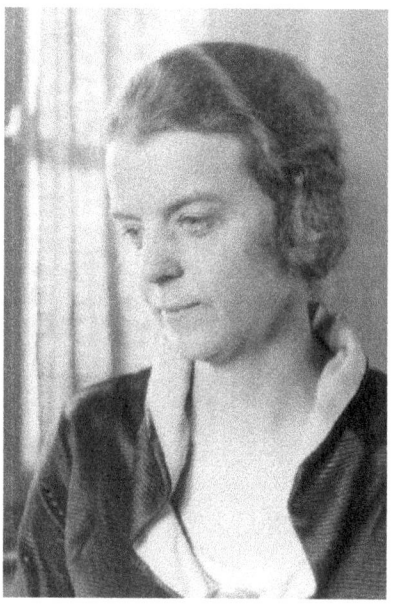

Martha Hemsoth, Jan 29, 1887 – March 31, 1936

We have a great need for speech formation lessons from someone who has not just studied speech artistically, but who has a grasp of the whole science of it. I could find no-one better suited than you, dear Frau Hemsoth, because you can stand before us in freedom; you have mastered the art of speech, and at the same time have the capacity for insight into pathological conditions and possible means of healing.

    Ita Wegman to Martha Hemsoth

Martha Hemsoth

Dietrich von Bonin

The following account of how Martha Hemsoth, who was a singer, found her way to speech formation as a therapy is based on her correspondence with Marie Steiner, Ita Wegman and others, and on an essay by the physician Madeleine Petronella van Deventer.[1] Apart from these sources, as well as an article by Martha Hemsoth herself and some speech exercises from her time at the Sonnenhof Children's Home in Arlesheim, no further traces of her life have come to light. What there is, however, gives a very clear picture of the destiny of this artist and therapist from her 37th year up to the time of her tragic death at the age of 49.

Martha Hemsoth's contact with the Clinical Therapeutical Institute in Arlesheim is well documented and begins with her time as a patient at the Institute in March and April 1924. She wrote to Ita Wegman on the March 12, 'my lack of appetite for the last 4–6 weeks compels me to undergo medical treatment now.'[2] She was admitted shortly afterward and the treatment was successful. She wrote on June 10 after her return to Hamburg, 'to tell you how well I have coped with the stresses of life since my return, as it has been an enormously stressful time. I sleep really soundly, am refreshed and cheerful in the morning, have a healthy appetite, and look forward to my meals.'

It could not be taken for granted that this treatment was going to be successful. Martha Hemsoth, after a healthy childhood and marriage in 1919 at the age of 32, suffered increasingly from low energy and gynaecological problems, which culminated in an operation in 1923. Those years were marked by a lack of appetite and decreasing energy and courage to face life.

In the same letter she also described her anthroposophical activity in Hamburg, where together with Dr Victor Thylmann she gave an introductory course:

I am happy to hope that our work together will be successful. After all, I have received and won so much energy and strength from you: physical, of the soul and of the spirit! Every day, straight after lunch, I go for an hour's rest. However I do not sleep; instead I use the time well to work on self-knowledge.

From a letter to Marie Steiner of August 28, 1924 we learn about Martha Hemsoth's previous activity as an opera singer, about a problem with her voice, and Rudolf Steiner's ability to help even an experienced opera singer by means of a few telling suggestions.

She travelled to Arnhem for the great summer conference with Rudolf Steiner, where from 17–24 July 1924 he gave three concurrent lecture courses: an education course of nine lectures, Human Values in Education; 'The Karma of the Anthroposophical Movement' (published as Karmic Relationships Vol. 8); and three public lectures on medicine, 'What Can the Art of Healing Gain Through Spiritual Science?' (published in The Healing Process). In the last three lectures Steiner ranges from a concise description of the path into the spiritual world through a strengthening of the forces of thinking, feeling and the will, to a description of the threefold nature of the human being, from which he draws indications for certain anthroposophic preparations, including Bidor and mistletoe therapy. In each lecture he speaks particularly warmly about the Clinic in Arlesheim and his colleague Ita Wegman. In the members' lectures on the Karma of the Anthroposophical Movement, he brought themes to the Netherlands from the recent Christmas Conference in Dornach, this time mainly concerned with the working of the Michael impulse.

Martha Hemsoth took Mien Viehoff, who had fallen ill, back home to stay with her after the conference, and they remained friends for the rest of Hemsoth's life.[3] Besides the huge number of 17 lectures in eight days, and without regard for his already weakened forces, Rudolf Steiner took time to give effective advice to individual members:

After returning here from Arnhem, I naturally began at once to practise singing in the way Rudolf Steiner had advised me. Imagine my joy when after a few hours of practice I was able to sing the long aria from Aida, as well as Isolde's song as she died of love. And I must admit that before singing these pieces I had always been really anxious. One is always amazed by Rudolf Steiner's judgment and wisdom.

At the beginning of this letter, she applied for the Speech and Drama Course in Dornach which was to begin a few days later, from September 5 to 23, 1924. It left a deep impression on her which was to change her life.

In her earliest surviving letter to Marie Steiner (July 17, 1920) Martha Hemsoth had already told her of the founding of an Art Group in Hamburg, as well as her interest in contributing her artistic intentions — fructified by anthroposophy — to the life of culture, 'it should really be the case that all branches of art are cared for, as we saw done in an archetypal way at the Munich mystery dramas.'

From this reference we may infer that she was present at one of the performances of the mystery plays in Munich (1910–1913), and that by her mid-twenties she was already at home in the circle of committed anthroposophists.

In the middle of May 1926, at the age of 39, the singer learned at an audition with the director of music at the Hamburg Opera, after she had not sung on stage for seven years, that her voice had become too weak for opera, but that it would still manage concerts. Depressed, she reported this to Ita Wegman next evening, 'I went home in a state of distress, asking over again, "Destiny, what are your plans for us?" No answer came.' (Letter of May 15, 1926.)

The letter continues with an idea she had had to travel to the United States with her husband — also at a turning point in his professional life — and help to build up the work begun by Gracia Ricardo.[4] At the same time she intended to bring the impulses of the Speech and Drama Course to America: 'I too must go over there and develop what Dr Steiner gave in his drama course.'

The letter refers to a karmic turning point in Martha Hemsoth's life and closes with the intention to devote herself to spreading the content of the Speech and Drama Course. Owing to pressure of work, Ita Wegman did not reply personally but gave this task to her close colleague Mien Viehoff, also an artist and very likely a friend of Martha Hemsoth since the 1924 Arnhem conference.[5]

Viehoff wrote on 27 May, rather coolly, that the American project was completely based on itself, only working for itself. The passage closes significantly: 'As I said, Dr Wegman has unfortunately nothing to say in this regard.'

Nothing is known of any further involvement in this matter by the Hemsoths. The letter goes on to offer the important advice — should she (Martha) be determined to give shape to what Rudolf Steiner gave in the Drama Course — that she should get in touch with Marie Steiner, 'because that would have to be preceded by a training in speaking.'

This answer of Mien Viehoff's surely put the damper on enthusiasm for the America project, yet closed with the exhortation to build up something similar, however much effort it takes.

Martha Hemsoth had to be in the Clinic in Arlesheim once more from

October 23, 1927 until January 22, 1928, after being in good health in the interim. Her condition was similar to how it had been in 1924 and was treated similarly, following Rudolf Steiner's original indications, as revealed by her case notes in the Ita Wegman Archive.

During her stay at the Clinic, or possibly afterward, conversations apparently took place with Ita Wegman about the impulses arising from the Drama Course. On September 19, 1929 Hemsoth wrote to Wegman:

> I am choosing this way to tell you that last Tuesday I had an audition with Marie Steiner and can report that it really was a success all the way through. Frau Doktor was very amiable and showed extraordinary interest during and after the audition. She worked with me straight away for an hour and gave me advice for working further by myself. She said that she was sorry but she would be travelling for some time after Michaelmas with all her good colleagues, so I would only be able to have lessons there from the beginning of November. Then Frau Dr Steiner added that I should have a look at the part of the Guardian of the Threshold and give it my attention; she herself would like to go through it with me on her return. She found me more suited to the role than the present incumbent, as my voice had potential for a greater range of register and modulation. The musicality of my speech would also be very suitable for speaking for eurythmy. Of course I would have to study hard. I must view it as a great sign of trust that Frau Doktor said all that without reservation. I really wanted to tell you all this, as you are the instigator of it all. Please regard all of this as a personal communication. I am very grateful to you for starting me on a path which I am taking so gladly and which it seems to me that I am karmically bidden to follow.

On the one hand she was realizing an impulse which had its beginning half a seven-year phase earlier, after the unsuccessful attempt to begin a stage career once more; on the other Ita Wegman is identified as the companion of this decision. The prospect arises of a change from being a patient to becoming a colleague. Whether Marie Steiner's idea of putting Hemsoth in the role of the Guardian of the Threshold in the mystery play was ever attempted or realized is not known. The surviving records tend to point to the contrary.

Nearly a year later, on September 3, 1930, Martha Hemsoth reported happily from Freiburg to Ita Wegman:

> So this is where I've got to!! I've just received word from the
> leader of the branch here that he has heard from Marie Steiner
> that I am taking over the courses in speech formation here.
> Marie Steiner has also sent me a message to this effect. I will
> start teaching in the middle of the month ... I have to remember
> gratefully that it was you, Dr Wegman, who gave me the impetus
> for the first steps in this new phase of my life. I will do my best to
> make all my further steps worthy of that impetus.

In order to put this news in the right context, one needs to bear in mind that in those days an organized speech training had not yet developed. Students were taught by different trained colleagues under the close supervision of Marie Steiner for as long as seemed necessary. At the right time they were authorized to teach, that is they received a certificate attesting to their competence to teach and represent speech formation independently.

On the basis of her previous artistic and singing training and her strict discipline in practising, she attained this goal about a year after her audition with Marie Steiner. From the short essay by Dr Madeleine van Deventer on Hemsoth's life we may infer that she had already had lessons in Hamburg and Freiburg with trained speech artists, which is not chronicled in the correspondence with Ita Wegman.

> The significance of the word for healing was probably always
> clear to Ita Wegman — including the word spoken in the right
> way by the patient themselves, as it works back onto their own
> organism. With the situation in the Anthroposophical Society at the
> time, collaboration with those trained in speech formation at the
> Goetheanum was almost inconceivable.
>
> Then came the meeting with Martha Hemsoth, a member
> from Hamburg. She was an opera singer. One day (presumably
> in 1927) she decided to learn speech formation and took lessons
> in Hamburg with Frau [Margarete] Kugelmann. Marie Steiner
> encouraged her, and Günther Sponholz was her teacher in
> Freiburg in 1928 and 1929. Frau Hemsoth received her diploma
> at the beginning of the 1930s and gave a recitation evening at the
> Goetheanum. Soon afterward she began her work with speech
> formation at the Clinic. She worked with many patients and also
> with the physicians. Her workplace was a little-used conservatory
> in the garden behind the clinic.[6]

Van Deventer was presumably unaware of some of the details of what led up to this decision, which we are able to trace in the correspondence between Ita Wegman and Martha Hemsoth. On the other hand, the essay gives a first-hand account of Hemsoth's activity and is an invaluable document for her activity as a therapeutic speech practitioner. The prelude to Martha Hemsoth's actual activity with therapeutic speech came in a letter to her by Ita Wegman on April 28, 1931, which at the same time sheds a particular light on Wegman's ideas about therapeutic speech and what she expected of it:

> But I wanted to ask you something else as well. Some of our physicians, as well as the curative educators, have a great need for speech formation lessons from someone who has studied speech in such a way that not just the artistic comes to the fore, but that the whole science of it is included. ... I could find no-one better suited than you, dear Frau Hemsoth, because you can stand before us in freedom; you have mastered the art of speech, and at the same time have the capacity for insight into pathological conditions and possible means of healing. As someone who has been through an illness, you will have the necessary understanding for conditions of illness.

On May 1, Martha Hemsoth gave a positive answer to the enquiry: 'After due consideration I have come to the conclusion that I can take on the responsibility of accepting your request ... I have also written to Frau Dr Steiner that I would like to follow this request, hoping that she will be in agreement.'

This decision marked the start of a short, though intensive and fruitful, therapeutic speech activity with physicians and patients at the Clinic, co-workers at the Sonnenhof Children's Home, and also at Lauenstein, where she worked with numerous adult patients and probably also with children. She also travelled to the recently acquired Hamborn Institute, where she produced theatre performances. In Arlesheim she took on the artistic shaping of the festivals. On October 1, 1932 Ita Wegman wrote in reply to a letter that is lost:

> I have received your letter, in which you write to me about the performance you are planning in Hamborn. In the meantime I have also heard from Herr Pickert[7] who writes that the performance of Gryff the Bird was splendid. I cannot tell you how much that pleases me and how grateful I am to you for doing that. We would be happy if you would like to come here next week. We could then

perhaps firm up some plans for the future ... on Tuesday I could certainly be there for you and would be pleased to have another detailed lesson with you.

The last sentence documents Ita Wegman's interest in artistic speech formation, and also in furthering her own competence in a medium whose strength she wanted to experience and understand herself. Apparently she had lessons with Martha Hemsoth on various occasions, among other reasons as preparation for holding the Class Lessons.[8] This could by no means be taken for granted, given the alienation between those active mainly around Marie Steiner in Dornach and Ita Wegman and the circle round her. What the situation here demonstrates is how clearly Ita Wegman and Marie Steiner were able to separate personal difficulties from their awareness of the task and spiritual content of speech formation.

Two letters from Hemsoth to Wegman from the following years up to 1936 have been preserved. On March 28, 1934 she sent Easter greetings from Altefeld and reported on work at Lauenstein (the Lauenstein Curative Education Institute for Children with Special Needs Association was founded in 1924; in 1932 it moved from Jena to a former stud farm in Altefeld near Eisenach):

> At the end of last week the children had their end-of-term festival and one had the impression that very diligent work is being done with the children and that something is being achieved. In future the forming of speech should also be cultivated here intensely. This would be extremely beneficial for many of the children ... It is not exactly easy being in this secluded forest, far from where the Annual General Meeting is taking place just now!

Martha Hemsoth also laid a seed for 'the forming of speech' here (alongside Hamborn and the Sonnenhof) where curative education was put into practice. At the same time she experienced it as a burden not being able to be present at the Annual General Meeting to support Ita Wegman or mediate between the ever more strongly polarizing forces in the Anthroposophical Society. As is known, this polarization came to a head a year later in 1935 when Ita Wegman and Elisabeth Vreede were excluded from the Council of the Anthroposophical Society. We can only guess how painfully Martha Hemsoth, who was dedicated to Marie Steiner's speech impulse and at the same time working in the circle around Ita Wegman, must have felt this split.

Van Deventer wrote in her essay about this period:

A highlight of her activity was the production of The Sacred Drama of Eleusis by Edouard Schuré with the co-workers at Hamborn in 1935 ... In Arlesheim she also took on the artistic forming of our festivals. Her working with us was a great advantage for us all.

A letter from a pupil, who wrote to apologize for being late, documents Martha Hemsoth's therapeutic empathy:

I can no doubt tell you that your teaching means release from many years' torment and agony from which around 25 or 26 doctors were unable to liberate me, as they did not understand what was wrong with me. From this you may judge how dear and important to me the sessions with you are, and how grateful I am ... And I am looking forward so much to being able to live and work like a normal human being one day without having to make all sorts of concessions as I do to my colleagues and superiors at work for example. Dear Frau Hemsoth, I thank you with all my heart for helping me [become free] from being seen as half an idiot. That is exaggerated — but — one ought to exaggerate, oughtn't one, as that is how one learns to be moderate.

In order to understand Martha Hemsoth's last letter, which is undated but can be placed in its right order, reference needs to be made to another report by van Deventer, who wrote:

At the beginning of May [1934], Ita Wegman became ill ... Her fever was not very high, but increasingly took on a septic character. The course of the illness gave us more and more concern. We decided on a change of air.[9]

Ita Wegman then spent some weeks in the Swiss mountains. Although she regained strength she could not yet decide to return to Arlesheim. So she decided on a journey to Palestine, which she undertook in the company of close friends. After the strenuous days in Palestine she recovered for a few weeks on Capri, where van Deventer met up with her, and later travelled on to Rome.

Van Deventer continued her report on the lengthening convalescence after Wegman's critical illness: 'The co-workers in Arlesheim expected of me that I would gradually be able to move Dr Wegman toward returning home. It was not so simple.'

Judging from Hemsoth's letter, Ita Wegman must have included yet another halt in the gradual approach to the north side of the Alps, for Hemsoth reports on the cool breeze off the lake in Cannero, a small town on Lake Maggiore, from where van Deventer and also Hemsoth must have returned, still without Ita Wegman. Whether Hemsoth had already joined the group round Ita Wegman in Italy, possibly with van Deventer on Capri already or later in Rome, cannot be ascertained. In any event Hemsoth wrote from Arlesheim, immediately after her return, to Ita Wegman in Italy:

> Many thanks again for all the beauty that I was able to see and enjoy with you and through you. After you had gone, I sat down at the quay in the shade and quarrelled with the god Mammon who has so much power. But then I thought of what I need to care for, which I do so gladly, and a joyful urge toward home took the place of the quarrelling. ... It was very hot in the train and, once arrived in Basle I found intense heat there too. This morning one perspired even while sitting still. ... Everyone, in the Sonnenhof as well, was happy to hear something immediate and authentic about you and were radiant when I told them that you were getting on so much better ... May the lake visit and the stay in the south mean that we can all greet you here in good health again at Christmas. That will be your Christmas gift to us. Wishing you everything dear, beautiful and good for the immediate future, your grateful Martha Hemsoth.

With these loving and grateful words Hemsoth's last preserved letter to Ita Wegman ends. The latter actually returned to Arlesheim after an absence of nine months. She inaugurated Christmas festival work, relating inwardly to her experiences around the events in Palestine. Hemsoth probably also took part in these evenings; they were ideal for further consolidating her inner connection with Dr Wegman's impulses.

No further details relating to Hemsoth are known for the following year. Most probably she continued her activity at the different places where she worked till a serious accident which brought her terrible suffering and after 10 days the end of her life at the age of 49. Dr van Deventer reported on the origin of the disaster:

> She had begun her work at the beginning of the thirties. On March 21, 1936 a terrible catastrophe took place. She was cleaning a dress with gasoline in the cellar of Kirchner House and had not noticed

that the door to the central heating room was open. The gasoline vapours exploded. Frau Hemsoth became a burning torch. She cried for help and felt her way up the cellar stairs. The gardener, who had heard her call for help, ran in, covered her in blankets and was able to smother the fire. Frau Hemsoth was taken to the clinic at once. However the burns were so widespread that there was only a slight hope of keeping her alive. Dr Wegman and her assistants nevertheless fought unswervingly for Frau Hemsoth's life. At the same time they knew that — even if she survived — her face would remain seriously damaged. This caused Dr Wegman to drive forward with great energy the plan which had been fostered for a long time for a branch in Ticino, so that she could have a secluded retreat for Frau Hemsoth where she could be protected from the stares of the surrounding world.

Frau Hemsoth died on March 31, 1936 — for her it was a release from terrible suffering. Dr Wegman suffered unutterably from the events ... She telephoned me almost daily in London where I was at that time standing in for Dr Nunhofer at 10 Kent Terrace for three months. She urged my immediate return — although I would hardly be able to be a help anyway. On my return it was all over. All I could do was be present for the cremation. This harrowing destiny also deeply moved the speech artists at the Goetheanum. Many came to the funeral, including her teacher Günther Sponholz. He and others offered Dr Wegman, through me, their help for the continuation of the speech work with the patients. In her deep shock, Dr Wegman was initially unable to take this up. There had been this deep relationship of trust with Frau Hemsoth. She herself had also done much work with Frau Hemsoth, for instance in preparation for reading the Class Lessons.

The plans for Ticino were continued. The same year Casa Andrea Cristoforo in Ascona was acquired and in Spring 1937 the first patients were admitted — one year after the death of Frau Hemsoth.

Thus ended Martha Hemsoth's life, abruptly and harrowingly. It was not vouchsafed her to see the fruits of her work, nor could others at first link on to the impulse which she began. This riddle of a caesura went to such an extent that towards the end of the twentieth century hardly any of the therapeutic speech practitioners remembered or even knew of Martha Hemsoth.

Ita Wegman had at first apparently really hoped to save Martha Hemsoth's life. Five days after the accident she wrote to van Deventer:

> It was really a horror for us, particularly because we did not know what the consequences for Hemsoth would be. It was really serious: large burns on the arms, hands, legs, back; her hair was burnt away and her face swollen with many small burns. Thank God she appears to have got over the shock, and the burns are recovering, so that we still hope that all will go well after all.

Her hope was not fulfilled, and we read in a letter of April 15, 1936 to Adam Bittleston:

> The death of our dear friend, Frau Hemsoth, has affected us all extraordinarily. We are all still deeply under the impression of this event. It will not be easy for us to fill her place, but we hope to be able to find the right person who can continue her work.

Van Deventer describes above why that did not happen. The exclusion of Ita Wegman and Elisabeth Vreede from the General Anthroposophical Society on April 14, 1935 was the final act in a process of increasing estrangement between Ita Wegman and Marie Steiner, described and commented on in detail in many places, which does not need to be outlined here.[10]

This event, which can hardly be understood from today's perspective, must have brought Martha Hemsoth great inner pain, as she had much gratitude and respect for both personalities. It was her particular destiny to have Marie Steiner's impulses deeply anchored within herself and then to place them as a fruit at the disposal of Ita Wegman's medical stream in selfless dedication. In this way she became a bridge-builder at a time when outer collaboration between the two streams was impossible for human reasons.

The circumstances surrounding Martha Hemsoth's death speak an earnest language. Only a few years after the fulfilment of a wish, which when looking at her biography appears as the real goal of her life, she was called out of her new life situation by a sudden accident. How many unfulfilled impulses must still have been alive in her which, however, might well not have reached fulfilment in the increasing darkening of Europe. Only a few years later, in 1939, another colleague of Wegman's, the physician Eugen Kolisko, died unexpectedly at the age of forty-six. And before the end of the Second World War Ita Wegman followed into the spiritual world at the age of sixty-seven, on March 4, 1943.

A decisive change and stabilization must have taken place in Martha Hemsoth's being during the few years' close collaboration as a therapeutic speech practitioner with Ita Wegman. Comparing the script in all her

28   THE BACKGROUND TO ANTHROPOSOPHICAL THERAPEUTIC SPEECH

earlier letters (1924–31) with that of the last letters from 1933 onwards, one notices a big difference. In the earlier letters a joined, sometimes nervous German handwriting prevails, flowing from the wrist, while the last letters are written more with unjoined, formed letters.
Extract from a letter, around 1928

Extract from a letter, 1934

Wegman's letter of April 28, 1931, decisive for destiny, speaks of three preconditions for working therapeutically out of the forces of speech formation, which today are just as relevant: first, mastery of the artistic means; secondly an eye for everything connected with conditions of illness and possibilities for healing; and thirdly an approach which is not only artistic but also scientific, which is not meant in the sense of evaluating, but relates to the necessary objectivity and reflection, which are essential for any therapeutic work.

Apart from the speech exercises and her letters, the only known written work by Martha Hemsoth is an undated essay on the mystery of effective speech. She writes here out of direct enthusiasm for the new forming of speech and its effectiveness on the listener, and less about the therapeutic effects. From its content, this essay would be placed in the period around 1929 and the intensive work with Marie Steiner, where it may also belong chronologically; that was the period in which she immersed herself completely in the artistic expression of the new speech formation.

What Martha Hemsoth wrote about speech at the end of the essay 'The Mystery of Effective Speech' became a reality for her:

> People [who dedicate themselves to it] will soon feel how they are strengthened in their personality, since hindrances of all kinds disappear, how they go through a process of healing, and learn to reach out with their personal forces through the word shaped in the flowing breath, speech formation.

Speech exercises

MARTHA HEMSOTH

The following exercises[11] by Martha Hemsoth for use with people with special needs rely in some cases, right down to the wording, on different speech exercises of Rudolf Steiner's. Presumably it was one of her concerns to make Rudolf Steiner's texts, which are consciously kept meaningless, into sentences more accessible to her clients.

Bleib bei biedern Bauern
Wenn wilde Wolken wuchten
Und blanke Blitze blenden

Griesgram, Griesgram, grauer Wicht,
Pack Dich, troll Dich, komm nur nicht
In meinen grünen Garten.

Dort im fernen Wüstenland
Da traben Tag um Tag
Drei beladne Dromedare.

Fern von Finsternissen
Fliegen feurige Vögel
Schwingen schwere Schwalben
Folg auf festen Füssen

Goldumglänzter grosser Gott
Gibst gern gute Gaben

Himmelshelle hoch und her
Sendet hold hernieder
Heilgen Hymnensang
Jedes Jahr jetzt jagen

Kühne kräftge Kerle
Jubelnd junge Junker

Kommt, kurze Kerle
Kräftge Knaben kommt,
Kantet kühne Keile
Keile kühne kantet

Lappige Lurche lieblich und leicht
Lallen wohl Lieder im lustigen Teich

Machtvollen Mut männiglich mehre
Menschliche Milde mässge Übermut

Nur nicht nörgeln und sich winden,
Man muss mutig Missmut bannen.

Pfiffig pfeife pferche Pferde
Pflege Pflänzchen pfropfe Pfirsiche

Protzig preist Bärbchen Banbo
Poltert putzig bei dem Bückling
Purzelnd pustend bricht das Beinchen

Rolle Rädchen rolle
Rund herum nur rase
Rase nur herum im Rund

Sanftes Säuseln seligen Wesens
Sänftigt sachte Stürme und Streit

Schlange zischt im Busch
Scheuch sie schnell husch husch

Tue tüchtige Taten
Taten tüchtige tue
Tätigkeit ertüchtigt

Weia wage, woge Du Welle
Walle zum Weltmeer
Wagala weija
Wehen Winde, wuchten Wolken

Wolken wuchten, Winde wehen
Wollend wirken Weltenwesen
Weltenwesen wirken wollend

Xaver Xenien dichtet x-beliebig lang
Xylophon auch spielt er x-beliebig lang

Zuboden zwingen zwar
Zehn zweckige Zwacker auf einmal
Zwanzig Zwerge zu Hanf

The mystery of effective speech

Martha Hemsoth[12]

Demosthenes was held to be the greatest orator of the Greek world. A power of the word proceeded from him which kindled and shook the souls of his listeners and enthused them to great deeds. It is reported that Philip of Macedonia feared the speeches of Demosthenes more than the armies and fleets of the Athenians.

One knows that the human being can be affected through the spoken word in a way that is quite impossible to describe. This power of the word becomes a mystery for modern human beings. They know neither its origin nor its being. Every speaker would like to possess it, but only very few are given the power of the word. Most people speak ineffectively, and even when they have to give speeches day in, day out, they may grow into the routine of guiding their thoughts, but seldom into the power of the word. People today generally do not believe that one can acquire this power. Yet there are ways to it.

History tells us that Demosthenes had a complete failure with his first speech. He spoke with long, winding, compound sentence structures and indistinct articulation, and was short of breath. He had to leave the stage amid booing and hissing. His friend, the actor Satyros, took on the quite demoralized Demosthenes and made him aware of the mysteries of eloquence. He practised tirelessly to bring about the right shaping of the word and an enlivening of speech, with the result that a person who was not gifted at speaking became the greatest orator of Greece, and 'world-famous' in that time.

Where is the mysterious power through which the human being is able to form the word so effectively? It is easy to understand that it does not arise from the content alone. How many excellent thoughts are spoken by speakers, professors, teachers or ministers of religion, which die away without effect, bore the listeners, and do not enter into them. Only the rightly formed word does that and makes speech effective. The unique thing in effective speech is that it not only works on the intellect but takes hold of the listener in their heart, takes hold of their will and penetrates into the depths of their personality. The Greek historian, Dionysius of Halicarnassus, in his treatise, On the Admirable Style of Demosthenes, shows that the secret of the demonstrative, overwhelming might of those speeches lay in the fact that they kindled all the feelings of which the heart is capable: 'One emotion after the other possesses the soul; suspicion, interest, fear, contempt, hatred, pity, good will, anger, jealousy: the totality of all the emotions that can storm the mind awake in me, when I hear the speeches of Demosthenes.'

A thought which is expressed only 'thoughtfully' does not work into the depths of what is human. The bridge which connects the speaker and the listener is made by the breath. But the breath with which the human being usually speaks is short, powerless and unable to carry the Word, empowered by the 'I', over to the listener. The normal way of speaking relates to speech that is developed and formed in the breath as oscillations in the air caused by noises comparable to those brought about by musical tones.

The effectiveness of speech lies in that the speaking human being (speaker or actor) is able to shape his words into the breath; that the breath itself is formed and thereby gains real strength and ability to carry to the listener the soul and spiritual forces going out from the speaker.

Only few human beings today have this artistic power of speech 'formation'. Those who have not received such a gift through destiny, or only insufficiently, can only instil it into themselves through training. They must work on themselves consciously, under the guidance of persons who know about it.

And it is very important that that happen; for good speaking is not merely an essential precondition for personal success, but it is a necessity of general significance. Today one realizes far too little what, for instance, a teacher without energy, which means speaking purely thoughtfully without heart forces, brings about in the souls of the children. Children seek eagerly for human contact; they are disappointed when a teacher only speaks to them intellectually. They suffer something then which is as if they were being dried out in their soul. Adults suffer something similar when they have to let the purely intellectual, powerless speech of their fellow human being wash over them.

Really speaking to the human being, effectively and artistically, is closely connected with the development of social forces. This art, which was practised extensively in antiquity, has to be acquired again today. People will soon feel how they are strengthened in their personality, since hindrances of all kinds disappear, how they go through a process of healing, and learn reach out with their personal forces through the word shaped in the flowing breath, speech formation.

Hildegard Jordi

A BRIEF AUTOBIOGRAPHY[1]

Born January 18, 1908 in Bowil, Switzerland — died August 8, 1998 in Münsingen, Switzerland

I grew up as the only child of teachers called Jordi-Kallen in Uetendorf (near Thun, Switzerland], which was then still a small, quiet farming village.

My mother, who loved her profession, practised it with great devotion and a well-developed sense for what is genuine and true and for what is right educationally. Her goodness and warmth of heart shone through my childhood like a sun, and her strong, upright being gave me security and purpose.

My father worked as a mathematics teacher at the secondary school. He was a Goetheanist: in all that he did, he took his departure from the matter at hand; in this way he developed in his students a living and independent way of thinking that was close to life. He awoke the need for clarity: everything had to be in the right place, one aspect arising from another. Through this way of teaching, which was marked by a developed sense of responsibility and an infectious enthusiasm, he created foundations which stood me in extremely good stead later when meeting anthroposophy.

I was happy in the simple conditions of the village and my family. My parents loved and valued me. I felt secure in their midst.

The only shadow which lay over my otherwise carefree childhood was my weak health. A bronchial condition from birth hindered me so much that I was never able to easily take part in games and sport. As a result I was a child who possessed little stamina and, from an early age, had to forego those things that my contemporaries were able to enjoy.

This was most painfully so later at the time of choosing a profession. My great and only wish was to study medicine. Our family physician who, for the reasons I have given, was firmly convinced that my health would not be up to the demands of a profession as physician, advised against it so decisively that my parents agreed with his conviction and would not allow me to study medicine. They thought a profession as teacher would be the most appropriate solution. Resigned to this and deeply downcast, I gave in to their will and entered the Monbijou seminar in Berne in Spring 1924.

I experienced the materialistic worldview, into which I was immediately led there, as an attack on my feeling and thinking. My endeavour to disprove what was laid before me in clear proofs failed ever more. In this way my previous completely whole world began to collapse on itself. Cold meaninglessness, emptiness, nothingness drew their threatening circles ever more closely about me — the fall into the abyss would probably have been unavoidable had music, as a messenger of heaven, not given its divine blessing.

From my ninth year on I had piano lessons. When I was introduced to Bach's Well-Tempered Clavier as a child, a redeeming world began to open up in me, which nourished and carried me during the time of my training and later when I worked as a teacher. Music remained my only real relationship to the divine, spiritual world up until my meeting with anthroposophy. I experienced in a wonderful way the first awakening to the meeting with Rudolf Steiner through my piano teacher Willy Burkhard. He challenged me to become a performer of Bach, whereupon the meaning and goal of my life lit up for me in a flash: yes, that is what I want!! But I want to do it out of new forces.

Out of new forces — what were they, and where were they to be found? ... I sensed that someone really great must be connected to these 'new forces'. Yet where was he and how was he to be found?

An indescribably deep longing came over me, and the belief began to grow that he or his work would take hold of me and bring me great fulfilment. This fulfilment was granted me, suddenly, with hugely convincing power, at the last place where I sought it — the Goetheanum in Dornach. I sat there one day, as if washed up by chance, to see the complete performance of Goethe's Faust, weighed down by preconceptions and not prepared to take it in with sufficient positivity.

But the 'Prelude in the Theatre' surprised and gripped me. This was drama as I had never before experienced it: grand, genuine, true, bubbling over with life, healthy — archetypally healthy! My involvement and deep feeling grew from scene to scene, until in 'Forest and Caves' I suddenly experienced 'these are the new forces which were awakened in me through Willy Burkhard and so deeply longed for ever since.' Like a fanfare this direction into the future tore me out of the dust of my downfall. At last, at last, I had found my true, spiritual home. After I had broken the old circle of my life and left it, and had been accepted into the training class for speech formation and theatre, my great wish to become a pupil of Kurt Hendewerk was soon fulfilled.

As the actor playing Faust he had brought me enlightenment as to my destiny. It had also become clear to me that this was the person I wished to train with. My time as a pupil lasted many years and was decisively significant for my existence then and in the future.

Among all the other personalities who nurtured my artistic development at the Goetheanum, I have to thank above all Edwin Froböse, Gertrud Redlich and Lea van der Pals.

Rudolf Steiner is said to have called the Goetheanum the House of the Word. That is surely what it was for all who experienced in it the power of speech that could work wonders — festivals of the spirit, which were received in deepest gratitude and which kindled the wish to remain connected with this stage for all of one's life.

I believed myself near to this lofty aim, when Frau Marie Steiner, who always worked very intensively with me, worked in a rehearsal with me on the role of the Guardian of the Threshold once more and on our taking leave of each other sent me off with the words: 'you need the opportunity to play big roles.'

I was all the more bewildered when Kurt Hendewerk, who also directed, said to me shortly afterward that he would not be able to give me any more big parts unless my health improved. In such cases there is often only one thing that helps: a year of recuperation in one's homeland. 'Do this! I hope you will return strengthened.'

For the first time since becoming his pupil the ground gave way beneath me ...

The doctor I visited was honest. He told me quite frankly that my bronchial tubes were too small and weak, and that nothing could be done as it was hereditary. I knew then that the year's renunciation that had been demanded of me had to be taken as the permanent closing of a portal. That was hard, shatteringly painful. I arrived at my parents' house like a castaway. Everything seemed lost and despairing.

Then a ray of light suddenly shone into my darkness — I could hardly believe it. On behalf of Professor Friedrich Eymann I was asked if I would give speech formation sessions in a course for teachers. I joyfully agreed.

I knew Professor Eymann very well, held him in high esteem and respected him. During my time in Dornach in many conversations he had suggested what I should read in literature, philosophy and anthroposophy. I was able to approach him with all my questions in these areas, and from his comprehensive, wonderfully profound knowledge he gave me very valuable suggestions. He often gave lengthy introductions to the works which he recommended to me for study.

His teaching gave me the direction I needed and complemented the artistic training provided by the Goetheanum. So when the course mentioned above had finished it was a great honour that he wished to include me in the anthroposophical courses which he had founded. (The basis for this was the request from many of the course participants to continue with the introduction to speech formation.)

Work with all these gifted and open people was very interesting. We were enlivened, refreshed and invigorated. However the awakening, formative power of the word and of speech formation soon entered areas that were problematic. Many students had karmic issues that had not been dealt with, or outer difficulties; these needed to be resolved urgently and called for a new direction in my work.

As some deeply depressed people were also in touch with me then, the call to develop new therapeutic speech methods became ever louder.

Rudolf Steiner developed eurythmy therapy (therapeutic eurythmy) as well as artistic eurythmy. Something analogous for speech formation was not given. He only indicated that in the word, the breath and in the methods of speech formation great healing forces were to be found. As he was not able to give a therapeutic system, those of us who were active in speech formation had to elaborate it.

The proficiency I had achieved and the opportunity to continue working with Kurt Hendewerk gave me not only courage for the venture but also hope that it would be possible to open up this new area of therapy.

I worked in this way for over thirty years and experienced how urgently our time needs this work. The word and the practice of speech formation are great aids for leading toward self discovery and inner harmony. This has proved itself under very different conditions and with differing developmental potentials. Because the threshold between a healthy and unhealthy life of the soul is fluid, soul therapy and work in education and development interweave.

Through devoting myself to attempts to resolve these problems, I experienced the deepest joy and, in a wonderful way, the guidance of destiny in my life: my heart bled when I had to forego the practice of medicine. Through meeting anthroposophy and the speech formation training, there opened up for me possibilities for healing which corresponded much more closely with my inner being and the state of my health. Art, which I had experienced since early youth as the very element of my life, now became the creative source of my work instead of science.

So this review of my life is filled with deep gratitude for the divine guidance which brought me this fulfilment.

Therapeutic methods for psychiatric illnesses

Hilde Jordi

The rapidly growing number of people who are mentally ill is one of the most urgent problems of the present. People are becoming ill from the hectic pace and the repelling technological coldness of our time.

When Hilde Jordi first told me of her work with people with psychiatric disorders, I was greatly surprised. Here was something new, which did not come out of psychiatry, which approached the illness with a completely open mind and helped these people to find themselves again.

This almost playful way of approaching the client and then exploring with them and dissolving the depths of their despair is impressive. It is a necessary addition to existing psychotherapeutic methods.

Peter Walser, MD

My path to psychotherapy proceeded out of purely artistic endeavours: I wanted to become an actor and, as I was deeply impressed by the performances of Goethe's Faust at the Goetheanum in Dornach, I decided to take the acting training established there.

Shortly after the end of my training I was asked to take on the introductory drama course in a week-long workshop in anthroposophical pedagogy.

Although this task lay far from the aims to which I aspired, it aroused my interest and later my complete commitment. Among the many participants I noticed some whose features were etched with suffering and who aroused my compassion. It soon became apparent that they were depressed and unable to respond to the way I worked with the others taking part. I therefore felt I had to tailor my approach to their state of mind, which was new to me. This seemed to go really well, and I soon noticed that a fleeting inner invigoration became perceptible in certain of these suffering souls — an outcome which filled me with a joyful sense of gratitude, for it hinted at future attainments, and summoned me to an immediate and unconditional commitment.

At the end of the course thirty participants expressed their wish to continue with this work. They all wanted individual instruction, which brought the opportunity for an intimate response to their individual questions and difficulties. It soon became apparent that these were oppressive for a large part of my students.

As I had already noticed in the course sessions, they suffered from depression which was often so severe that they were hardly able to manage the demands of their occupations. The destiny of these unhappy souls touched my heart. I felt that I was not to shrink from the task they presented to me.

Working with people who have depression

In order to be as clear as possible, I will take a typical case of this kind. One of my students told me that he found it extremely difficult to discuss an issue or give a presentation on it. Even though he clearly understood the factual content, it was not possible for him to present his views or convictions in front of other people. He was so overcome by timidity and anxiety, which were baffling to him, that he had to break off before he had really started. He said this was terribly embarrassing for him and that he could not imagine how he could continue his studies in this state. He also suffered from depression which was becoming more and more unbearable, hindered him in his work and prevented him from sleeping. Ever more frequently he had to get up in the middle of the night and walk down to the lake ...

The seriousness of the situation was clear to me. The temptation to turn away this person who was in such peril, was great and seemed also to be the only right and responsible thing to do. And yet I could not do it. An inner admonition, that the courage would have to be found to strive toward new goals and seek new ways, became ever louder and more insistent — until suddenly an enormous power of trust in the ability I had achieved and in the conquering might of the spirit awoke in me. In this cathartic confidence the decision to risk the solitary, perilous journey into the unknown arose in my wrestling soul. As the speech exercises that I had introduced in the courses were of no further help, the necessary means had first to be created. A first stage paving the way had to be sought and established. But what could it be?

In the first lesson the young man's great introversion was already apparent to me. But what stood behind it? Was there a possibility to bring the dammed up forces into flow and turn them toward the world outside? How could a real relationship to it be schooled more fundamentally and archetypally than through speech?

Then the old children's games such as marbles and skittles occurred to me. Out of consideration for the other occupants of the house we substituted rubber balls for the wooden skittle ones. We then rolled them back and forth to each other. In this way the client was led back into the time before his illness — what was healthy could take hold of what was healthy — this proved a good place to start.

In order to continue training the relationship to the outside world in as living a way as possible, and for variety, balls, cushions and javelins were thrown. The javelin throwing was practised in the open air. When this was not possible, smaller sticks were thrown at a target in the practice room. Then rolling the ball at each other was accompanied with ri, ra, rutsch. I rolled the ball to the student with ri: he rolled it back to me with ri. Then the same with ra and rutsch.

When this exercise becomes a kind of agility game it has an excellent effect in that the urge to move awakens fully and the relation to the outer world can be schooled in a very fundamental way, until being happily active becomes a matter of course. The importance of movement in psychotherapeutic work could be experienced in an immediate and impressive fashion.

It was very important for continuing the work that movement should be consciously included with all speech formation activity. How this was done cannot be demonstrated and brought to experience through a mere description. Anyone who has ever seriously taken up artistic studies knows from experience that the most intimate and often the most essential matters can only be experienced and attained in immediate imitation (teacher–student). An example of this is the way in which the movement impulse takes hold of the sounds and the words and leads them into the space.

Because the teachers working psychotherapeutically see depression, apart from its aspect of suffering, as a condition of soul that is dammed up, immobile and inert, they find the way indicated — of bringing movement into the intonation of the sounds — as a great help which from then on proves immensely effective.

I will not be considering this aspect again in what follows. However it should still be included by the reader as a kind of undertone, an element that underlies everything.

The enlivening and strengthening effects of practising in this way were soon apparent. The young man's condition became more active. And yet, by comparison with many other people with depression who could genuinely be healed in the way described, this patient's condition, while certainly improved, was not yet fundamentally healed. A mysterious something stood in the way of all further efforts in this direction, impeding them.

At that time I was reading again the lectures on Speech and Drama which Rudolf Steiner had held in 1924. There I came on the passage where the temperaments are discussed. The following is a direct quote: 'We have the means at our disposal for evoking temperament, only we don't use them.'[1]

This indication has a power of kindling. It was the temperament that was completely lacking with this young man. This showed a marked discrepancy with his outer appearance which was strongly shaped in a choleric way. This is what I suddenly realized. The very promising prospect that suppressed temperaments could be freed gave me the necessary direction and confidence.

As the blown sounds stand in relation to the choleric temperament, I began practising with F F – S S – Sh Sh – Ts Ts and so on.

My student imitated me dully and without fire. In the belief that he did not dare show his temperament, I gave him a little sermon which culminated in an assertion that choler was a gift of God which melted all ice and victoriously opened up the way to hearts.

The hoped-for effect of my words did not come about. Renewed attempts with the exercises mentioned showed clearly that he was not able to go into this way of freeing the temperament. I therefore put my further hopes for a solution to the riddle in conversation. This happened and I learned the following.

Through his quick temper and fits of rage, a brutal and tyrannical teacher had scared the sensitive boy and made him anxious, so that he experienced himself as defenceless and abandoned, confronted by a force that was annihilating him. In his plight, from which there was no escape, the resolve grew to do all he could never to fall into such contemptible behaviour himself. Out of the intense indignation at the suffering that had come his way grew the strength to nip any signs of aggression in the bud and eventually also to suppress completely his mightily blossoming choler.

The growing youth was visibly proud of this deed, which had cost him so much; for the choler in his view was simply evil. If someone succeeded in suppressing it totally they would have saved the nobility of their soul and found peace with themselves and others.

This conviction was so deeply anchored that it took several conversations to be able to resolve on a transformation of it. There was also still a way to go to becoming grateful for the grace of this gift and its wonderfully enthusing quality.

However this way did not lead through the wasteland, because the pupil's perspective could now be expanded as he was led gently into the mysteries of the breath: opening himself in the in-breath, giving himself up to the experience of the sounds and words that were to be formed — then the interplay of reciting them in the outgoing stream of breath, which was experienced as a primal creative activity, and practised in an elemental way using hu hu hu.

This work directed more toward the spiritual pole was complemented by going into the physical function of the breathing: when one breathes in, the diaphragm is pressed down. If one has fully lived through the spiritual aspect described above, one experiences the following as the physical counter movement that is called forth: while the soul and spiritual soars upward, the physical strives to sink in and anchor itself, powerfully pressing down the diaphragm, thus preventing its being dislocated while in a state of relaxation.

It is a joy with an open-minded student to listen in to how nature has impressed into us an archetype which maintains equilibrium, balance and inner harmony. This knowledge has fundamental significance and reveals its usefulness to a high degree in therapeutic work .

With the young man, the movement of the diaphragm was wrong, as is the case with a great number of our contemporaries; so it was corrected and was checked in every lesson until the danger of falling back into bad old habits had been overcome.

The exercises with the blown sounds, which had been stopped, were now taken up again; one could clearly see that, thanks to the discussion mentioned above, the inner torpor was beginning to dissolve. This awoke the hope that along the path that was being followed the releasing of the choleric temperament would happen quite organically as of its own accord.

Now I turn to the other results of the so tragically misunderstood aims toward which my pupil had been striving: the soul was weak. Filled with anxiety and uncertainty, it had let itself be driven more and more into an ill-omened escape from itself.

As a boy he already gone out of the way of difficulties; as a growing youth he increasingly avoided conflict and competing with others. Healthy self-assertion and self-realization were not achieved. Because of this one had to reach out much further than had seemed necessary to start with. Because his inner life always tended to flow away and was wholly without contour, he first needed to acquire the capacity for consolidation. In speech, the young man lacked E, K and I. That is where a start had to be made and where we had to put all our energy into doing now what had been missed earlier. E E became the leitmotif of what we strove for together in the following lessons. It was at once apparent that opportunities missed in the past were very difficult to make good later. An intoned E was so lacking in energy and strength that it was hardly able to shape the soul. Situations calling for him forcefully to defend himself had therefore to be found. As an aid I took a text by Rudolf Steiner for eurythmy therapy:

> Ich wehre dir den Weg
> Ich wehre dir den Steg
> Ich helf mir selbst.[2]

> Defending the way
> Defending the stage
> I help myself.

As the content of these three lines is clothed within the gesture of the sound E, this verse soon revealed itself as the exercise which could not be bettered in its effectiveness.

We played soldiers as well. The soldier has to defend a pass: Ich wehre dir den Weg! [literally: I'll defend the path against you]. A new onslaught of the enemy had to be resisted: Ich wehre dir den Steg! [literally: I'll defend the footbridge against you]. Or we took hold of each other in single combat and tried to push back the enemy with: Ich helf mir selbst! [literally: I'll help myself]. The E was supported each time by the corresponding eurythmy therapy gesture.

Sometimes this went really well. Yet it was clear that the condition of my pupil was still too slack. He had still not managed to assert himself convincingly. The purely vocalic had now to be complemented by the addition of a consonant, in this case the K. Its sharply contoured force became the chisel which began to shape the mushy soul.

The image came to me of woodcutters from earlier times before mechanization (for example, Ferdinand Hodler's The Woodcutter). These rugged men of mighty strength who towered above purely intellectually trained gentlemen with university degrees became the ideal to be striven for. Their deeds were emulated: wood was split with the axe, the blow delivered accurately, forcefully and cleanly. It was most effective when the stiffly stretched-out right hand was experienced as the axe and made the cut powerfully.

After that the situation was changed. A strong personality (for example, a judge or a teacher) summons a delinquent before him: Komm Kerl! [come fellow!]. The two words beginning with K were supported by the blow with the right hand, in such a way that the gesture with the hand and the intoned words exactly coincided. This way of working had an excellent effect.

The summoning judge was then replaced by the 'educator' who had been experienced as the cause of the young man's developmental difficulties and was therefore bitterly hated as the arch-enemy. In order to give free rein to the pent-up thirst for revenge, we became Greek warriors. On the battlefield of the Iliad we strove resolutely to emulate those heroes, who lived beyond our ideals of morality.

To jettison for once the proper behaviour of our bourgeois society, which has long since been brought into question, and be allowed to erupt from the depths of the soul in a safe way, was an incomparable draft of health. A space arose which he could enjoy, a space of inner truth where that teacher was put in his place and given a good hiding; through this my pupil was able to win through to great inner liberation by vehemently giving vent to the power within.

In cases like this being given permission to express oneself from the depths of one's instinctual life can be of decisive help and can open the door to real healing.

Intensive guidance in out-breathing was connected with this breakthrough. In the nature of things, strong experiences call for powerful forming of the outward flow of the breath.

The breath exercises given by Rudolf Steiner were now required. I introduced them, and it was astonishing how quickly the breath became free and flowing. Receiving and giving away, those archetypal principles of experience and behaviour worthy of the human being, became more spontaneous and convincing.

Further exercises, some of which had already been worked on earlier, were now added. Emphasis was again placed on inner strengthening and on freeing the choleric.

The results were discouraging. Even though a certain strengthening was clearly perceptible, one still had to admit that efforts to liberate the choleric remained unsuccessful.

What was to be done? Since the revealing conversation had created a new basis, I believed it would be possible to take up once more the exercises with blown sounds. In vain. The more resolutely I aimed at solving the problem in this way, the more the solution eluded me. I wondered if I would ever be able to lift the veil of this mystery and be able to work cathartically on the heavily shrouded forces of the temperament.

One day, as I sat despondently on a bench in the garden after further fruitless efforts, staring into the impenetrable darkness of the nearby fir trees, my gaze fell on a cat creeping through the grass in front of me, which had apparently spotted a mouse — for it crouched down, tense and expectant, and began to swing its tail back and forth before suddenly coiling up for the well aimed pounce at its prey, which it caught and darted off with.

As if nature wanted to reveal her mystery to me, what I had seen leapt like a spark into my soul: that was it! It was by means of an inner coiling up that the repressed choleric temperament was to be awakened and set in motion.

A veritable storm of enthusiasm broke out within me. I rushed into the house and straight away began to live into what I had just seen, so utterly to become a cat that I was almost convinced that I could feel its tail and swing it to and fro. I believed I could experience the primeval excitement of a half-slumbering force from the depths which stimulated extreme tension.

That was a stroke of luck! I practised and practised and could hardly wait for the moment when I would be able to reveal this healing discovery to my student.

When at last he stood before me and I introduced the cat as his great inspirer and master, I realized to my great satisfaction that, after practising only briefly, the choleric temperament was beginning to appear. What I had so ardently hoped for had come about.

Now the arduous phase, in which the lost, instinctive awakening of the temperament had been tracked down, was over. The light of consciousness had been able to illumine the darkness. In our situation it was the secret, gleaned from nature, that the power of the choleric temperament had to be awakened. And since this arousing of the suppressed choler could not be brought about by the intellect, the image of the cat pouncing on its prey proved true to life, exactly corresponding to what was needed.

What still had to be done was to train the capacity that was to be acquired; for an instinct that has been lost cannot suddenly be restored to its original functioning by illuminating it with consciousness. Instead the capacity which is to replace it must be schooled consistently until it has reached an equivalent completely independent functioning. In terms of our practice this meant that the forming of the sounds, which with a suppressed temperament was sluggish and feeble, had to be practised in connection with the pounce of the cat until the activation of the choleric temperament took place as if of its own accord, thereby enabling the sounds to be intoned energetically and powerfully.

In order to avoid misunderstandings I must mention that when I say the pounce I do not just mean its culmination, but particularly the preparation leading up to this: the exact imitation of the cat's behaviour, the crouching down, and awakening the impelling power of the choleric temperament through excited movement while in this posture.

Exercises with initial blown sounds, which are directly related to the choleric, and appropriate texts were now drawn on. We proceeded in this way until to crown our efforts we worked on the following poem by Friedrich Hebbel.

Zu Pferd! Zu Pferd!

Zu Pferd! Zu Pferd! Es saust der Wind!
Schneewolken, düstre, jagen!
Die schütten nun den Winter aus!
Zu Pferd! Zu Pferd! Durch Saus und Braus
die heisse Brust zu tragen!

Mit krausen Nüstern prüft das Ross
Die Luft, dann wiehert's mutig;
Nur wie ich herrsche, dient das Tier,
Ein Druck: von dannen fliegt's mit mir,
Als wär mein Sporn schon blutig.

In meinem Mantel wühlt der Wind,
Er raubt mir fast die Mütze;
Ich hab ihn gern auf meiner Spur,
An seiner Wut erprob ich's nur,
Wie fest ich oben sitze!

To horse! To horse! The wind, it blows!
Dark snow-clouds are racing
And chasing the winter away!
To horse! To horse! To bear
My burning breast through rage and roar!

With flaring nostril the steed is testing
The air, then neighing mightily;
Only my rule will master the beast:
A touch — then away it flies with me,
As if my spur were bloodied already.

The wind is billowing in my cloak,
Near tearing away my bonnet;
I'm glad to have him on my heels,
Only his rage allows me to tell
How sure my seat here on high.

My student practised this now with great enthusiasm. He was able to find and experience an inner liberation and affirmation of himself in it. Someone disabled for years had found his way back to his being, gloriously fired with enthusiasm and rich with impulses. Borne by the reawakened forces of his inner life, he began to reach for new horizons.

We continued our work together in this vein for some time in order to consolidate what had been achieved.

The student completed his studies with distinction and with the best mark in the exam. Since then his achievements have been of the same standard. He has had no relapses.

I have attempted to show from the case described above how, from my point of view, I experienced the background and aetiology of the lack of motivation, inner uncertainty, timidity, anxiety and depression, and developed appropriate therapeutic measures. Over the years, thanks to greater experience, these could be applied more accurately. Essentially, however, they have not changed. Thus they have helped convincingly to show that a weakly developed or suppressed inner force can be awakened and schooled through the exercises described.

I should just like to add that the activities which had to be found through imagination, for example outbursts of rage against a traitor or learning to be assertive toward an overly authoritative teacher, were gleaned from the destiny which had not been mastered. In this way one did not simply practise blindly, but had a real confrontation with what tormented one and gave one the opportunity for inner growth.

Then a young man who had to suffer much at the hands of his despotic father, and who over a period of time used the sounds and exercises described to fortify and defend himself against him, came into the therapy session and exclaimed: 'Now I am saved! Yesterday I went up to my father for the first time and had the courage to tell him that it was high time he listened to me. I said I had subjected myself for too long to him and his opinion of me; now I wished to take up and carry out what I longed for and what I found appropriate. My father did not shout me down as he usually did, but listened to me and finally endorsed my plans for how I wished to conduct my life in future.'

With young and still quite impressionable people suffering from depression or who had no drive it was possible to bring healing or motivate them again in quite a short time, after a few lessons at the most. It took longer with middle-aged or older people. Here too, however, a complete cure or substantial improvement could also be achieved.

Bipolar affect disorder

After I had been working in this way for some time I was asked to take on a patient with bipolar affect disorder.

The patient had been having psychiatric treatment for two years and his physician welcomed my collaboration, as he hoped it would contribute to an enlivening of the patient's soul life.

In the initial conversation with the doctor he told me that the bipolar disorder had been so severe that he had found it necessary to sign him off from work two years previously. He was looked after by his parents and when in remission was able to help them in the garden or the household. When severely depressed he stayed in bed for days on end, and it was impossible to make demands on him such as a walk to the therapist.

When the young man first came to me, his depressive condition was immediately apparent. In order to get him out of this a little, I had him throw cushions and arrows and roll marbles and balls back and forth with me, as described above, as a transition into the E. He experienced the E as a powerful defence.

At the end of the session it was clear that the depression had lost some of its severity. The second session proceeded in a similar fashion.

He came to the third session in high spirits and was rather hyper. I tried to consolidate him with the E and draw him into his centre. In order better to connect his feet with the ground, I got him to do the eurythmic B with his legs. This helped so much that he finished the session in a basically normal condition.

This way of working continued for some time. Sometimes he was depressed when he came, sometimes manic. I always tried as far as possible to normalize him.

In the meantime I had had another conversation with the psychiatrist, in which he described bipolar disorder once more. He concluded by remarking that the patient had a thoroughly positive relationship to me, and that his changing dreams showed that my work was having a fortifying and enlivening effect.

I therefore continued in the same vein. I was unable to achieve substantial progress despite all my efforts — however I never lost my conviction that a decisive breakthrough might happen and lead to a turnaround.

I was therefore astonished when the psychiatrist asked me to meet him urgently. As soon as we greeted each other I could tell that something bad had happened. He said the following: 'Unfortunately it's not good news that I have to report. In spite of your help, there has been no decisive step toward curing our patient. I have taken all the measures at my disposal, but can now no longer take responsibility for treating him as an outpatient.

This means I will have to have him sectioned after all. He will have to spend the rest of his life in hospital. Admitting him like this will be the end of him.'

These words wounded me so deeply that I called out in despair, 'But doctor, I can see a way through! If you would give me the authority, I would like to try and rescue this poor soul.'

He consented, began to give me the reasons for his decision once more, and finally said very confidingly, 'I am not an anthroposophist. However anyone can see that anthroposophy is right at the forefront of curative education. What I have observed in this case leads me to hope that it will also be able to play a leading role in the field of psychiatry.'

I said goodbye and the door closed behind me. I suddenly halted as if rooted to the spot. An inner quaking came over me and I felt as though the burden would crush me.

When great new ideas fire our inmost soul, we are able to achieve extraordinary deeds without bothering to eliminate any associated risks. Breaking new ground leads us into dangers which we could never anticipate and which, even if we did recognize them, we would never wish to avoid.

Thus began this balancing act. It lasted for years and often led me to the edge of utmost despair. Yet my courage was fortified and fired again and again by the inmost conviction that I would continue to witness the healing power of the word, which I had experienced to such a high degree, and that I would attain the outcome for which I yearned.

When the young man came to me the following day I learned from him that the doctor had terminated his treatment. He thought this a good thing, as he had not been feeling comfortable for some time, but had complete confidence in the way we were working together.

I continued, in the way already described, what we had begun. A certain alleviation set in. The patient was more approachable and I soon discovered that he was able to carry on working inwardly with what we had achieved. This gave me confidence and courage.

As the depressive phase, through the experiences described at the beginning, was more approachable for me than the manic, I was able to stabilize the patient through a much deeper insight than was possible for me in the manic phase.

It became apparent to me that devoting myself completely to this difficult, apparently impenetrable field was my next urgent task.

I took as my starting point a speech exercise beginning with B: Bei biedern Bauern bleib brav (by beaten bowers bide brave). I intoned the B and the student carried it out with his legs in eurythmy in a very elemental way, completely involved like a prehistoric human being in the vigorous activity of his legs — being all leg, having to force a way through tall grass or undergrowth. This was practised until the joy and enthusiasm for this way of moving had overcome all the initial difficulties.

Then the bull was introduced: this colossus, rooted and anchored in the earth, was imitated. Learning to stand as firmly as he, so that nothing can uproot one. Remaining firmly grounded in any situation. Even when running not to lose connection to the ground. All of this was practised through imitation. The bull remained our instructor until we succeeded in standing in the meadow like him and, like him, were able to penetrate powerfully the earthly sphere and trustingly become part of it.

The more archetypally all this is experienced, the more stabilizing the effect. This activity was complemented by stepping rhythms backwards, to begin with exclusively trochees: long short — long short — long short. When manic tendencies were no longer apparent, the arms could be included, such that the backward step and the spreading of the arms coincided with the long. For a text we took Goethe's 'Ocean Stillness'. This poem is just right for such a situation; its greatness and artistic perfection can be felt in a wonderfully impressive way through an intimate hearkening to its inner order.

> Tiefe Stille herrscht im Wasser,
> Ohne Regung ruht das Meer,
> Und bekümmert sieht der Schiffer
> Glatte Fläche rings umher.
> Keine Luft von keiner Seite!
> Todesstille fürchterlich!
> In der ungeheuren Weite
> Reget keine Welle sich.

> Deepest stillness rules the water,
> Ocean rests without a stir,
> And the worried sailor looks on
> Smooth expanses all around.
> Not a breath from any aspect!
> Deathly stillness terrible!
> In the dreadful, spreading vastness
> Stir no wave nor billow now.

Each line was worked on separately. It was impossible to exhaust the potential of the following lines:

Tiefe Stille herrscht im Wasser,
Ohne Regung ruht das Meer,
Glatte Fläche rings umher.
In der ungeheuren Weite

We tried to get the forming of the stillness, the lack of motion, the smooth expanse and the dreadful vastness to flow through arms, hands and fingertips. Stepping into the lengths and filling them out of the experience of the smooth spreading of the arms, radiating calm, was a uniquely harmonizing activity.

Later we practised dactyls in a similar way: long short short — long short short with texts such as Schiller's 'The Dance':

Siehe, wie schwebenden Schritts im Wellenschwung sich die Paare
Drehen! Den Boden berührt kaum der geflügelte Fuss ...

See how with hovering steps, the couples like waves now are turning
Scarce do their feet touch the ground, moving as borne upon wings ...

Also individual lines from Goethe's 'Achilleis':

Hoch zu Flammen entbrannte die mächtige Lohe noch einmal,
Strebend gegen den Himmel, und Ilios' Mauern erschienen
Rot durch die finstere Nacht ...

Up blazed the flames of the mighty funeral pyre now once more
Striving on upward to heaven, the walls of Troy now appearing
Red through the dark, gloomy night ...

Through this way of working it was possible to counteract the bipolar condition from different angles. The outcome was gratifying. The upward and downward swings came less frequently and were less severe. This achievement filled me with the deepest gratitude; for the dangerous manic-depressive states and my attempt to approach them from my lonely standpoint had left their mark on me. Thanks to the improvement that had set in I could at last heave a sigh of relief and turn to other difficulties.

Foremost among these was the hardly improved lack of initiative, which is why I drew on exercises with blown sounds. Suddenly I realized how much the poor man still lacked fire and oomph. I found myself once more in the same situation as with the other student described at the beginning. Here also there was a strong disposition to the choleric, but totally suppressed. I therefore asked my client whether in the past he had been under the influence of someone who, as a result of his violent temper, had frightened or battered him. He described a tragedy that was so similar to that of the earlier student that I do not need to repeat it here. Even the reason for his suppressing his choleric temperament was the same as that of his fellow sufferer. For that reason I can go straight into my attempts to find a solution for this new set of problems.

As mentioned, a certain stabilizing of the bipolar disorder had been achieved; this encouraged me to begin liberating the choleric temperament by releasing and kindling it through practising blown sounds. As the patient appeared to be responding well, I encouraged his enthusiasm, until I suddenly became aware to my horror that I had propelled him not into the choleric but into mania.

Luckily I had just enough time before the arrival of my next student to bring him down again and stabilize him more or less before he left.

I was now confronted by a real challenge: while the tendency to get out of himself needed to be curbed or removed, the deep-seated but suppressed force within him needed to be awoken, kindled and liberated.

This failed attempt had made clear to me that the liberation of the choleric temperament might not be approached directly. It was apparent that the preconditions for such a bold approach were lacking and had therefore to be created.

It appeared to me that the urge to movement should form the point of departure, unsullied by any passionate elements, following only its own dictates, pure and chaste. Yet how could the way be found out of the patient's complicated and difficult inner condition to a state of paradisal innocence? Was there such a thing as an exemplar, and where was it to be found? This question occupied me much, but its solution came quite unexpectedly.

In the middle of a lesson, as I was guiding my pupil into movement in an enjoyable way, the image of a prepubescent child's delight in play came to me. The innocent devotion to movement, which characterizes play in early childhood in such a refreshing and divinely delightful way, provided just the example that I was looking for.

My pupil therefore had to imagine himself back in his early childhood. As he was by no means an insignificant individuality, he had a strongly developed sense for what was objectively right and a similar striving to put it into effect. He soon realized the higher significance of our apparently naive play and began to develop a very gratifying devotion.

I then took up once more rolling a ball back and forth with ri, ra, rutsch in the way I described earlier. I gradually increased the distance between us and increased the tempo so that, through the rolling activity in the room, his attention remained entirely on the breath. (I had thus come to the old children's games from a different angle to that in the earlier case.)

Practising this way had the great advantage that I could exactly observe the patient's state. A tentative ability to differentiate mania from a healthy manifestation began to become apparent, not only for the teacher but increasingly also for the pupil. This is of the greatest significance, for by practising so intimately and consistently not only is the soul strengthened but an inner capacity for orienting oneself is also developed.

The patient begins gradually to become aware of their tendencies to slip away from what is healthy and also acquires the capacity to overcome them. They begin to long for the joy of play belonging to early childhood and to need it more and more decidedly as an essential remedy. In this spirit it was necessary to build up this phase of inner development in such a way that it became a home for the soul and spirit in which a kind of basic orientation could be found at any time.

We practised further in this way and, after a certain assurance in what we were aiming at had been reached, were going to approach the blown sounds. Since these correspond in speech to the choleric temperament, it seemed necessary to safeguard the risky experiment as far as possible.

My pupil mounted his saddled horse (in his imagination), grasped the reins with his left hand (gesture of holding onto oneself), while his right hand, waving enthusiastically, seized and drove onward the syllables and words of the exercises and poems to be worked on.

In this way the curbing influence of the left hand could hold the manic tendency in check (the pupil was made to experience this fully); while through the exciting activity of the right the choleric temperament could be brought into full flow. To my great joy and satisfaction the attempt was so successful that it could be implemented as a future way of working.

In order to free the suppressed forces of the temperament more and more and bring them into movement, and in order to include a normal, fully human experiencing and reacting, I now began to work at individual lines or verses from appropriate poems.

The following verse from 'The Song of the Honest Man' by Gottfried August Bürger was very suitable:

>   Der Tauwind kam vom Mittagsmeer
>   Und schnob durch Welschland trüb und feucht;
>   Die Wolken flogen vor ihm her,
>   Wie wenn der Wolf die Herde scheucht,
>   Er fegte die Felder, zerbrach den Forst;
>   Auf Seen und Strömen das Grundeis borst.

>   From midday sea the thaw-wind blew

And Romandy dark and damp was riven;
The clouds before it fast they flew ,
As when the flock by wolf is driven.
It swept the fields, the forest crashed;
The ice on lake and stream it smashed.

Then we practised 'The Young Sailor' by Friedrich Hebbel in the same way:

> Dort bläht ein Schiff die Segel,
> Frisch saust hinein der Wind;
> Der Anker wird gelichtet,
> Das Steuer flugs gerichtet,
> Nun fliegt's hinaus geschwind.
>
> Ein kühner Wasservogel
> Kreist grüssend um den Mast,
> Die Sonne brennt herunter,
> Manch Fischlein, blank und munter,
> Umgaukelt keck den Gast.
>
> Wär' gern hineingesprungen,
> Da draussen ist mein Reich!
> Ich bin ja jung von Jahren,
> Da ist's mir nur ums Fahren,
> Wohin? Das gilt mir gleich!

The ship's sail is swelling,
The cool wind whooshes in;
The anchor is hoisted,
The rudder swiftly set,
Now swift be our flight.

A bold seabird,
Circling the mast, salutes;
The sun scorches down.
Many fish, shiny and jolly,
Splash brashly for the visitor.

I'd gladly have jumped in;
My empire is out there!
Because I'm young in years,

> It's all about the journey;
> To where? It's all the same to me!

All of this was practised in exactly the same way as was described above, namely up on horseback, with the left hand restraining and the right hand swinging the individual syllables onward.

It soon became apparent that the choleric temperament was beginning to be released from its repression and that the capacity to experience was also gradually coming to the surface. His facial features became softer, his gait and movements more flowing. This led me to hope that the methods developed to free the choleric temperament in the case of people with depression could also be implemented fully with this patient.

Unfortunately I had to admit that it was not possible to go beyond what had been achieved initially with the reined-back horse, as described above. What had gone really well in the therapy session, thanks to the therapist's supportive help, brought about dangerous confusion at home, where the patient was left to his own devices.

This showed clearly that the young man still needed my guidance in dealing with his pathological tendencies. And even though there was the prospect of his managing to deal with his problems by himself in the foreseeable future, the profound disturbances which accompany the complete liberation of the choleric temperament could not be risked now or possibly ever. These attempts were therefore broken off in favour of striving for the independence of his inner orientation in dealing with his pathological tendencies.

I believed I could stand behind this decision, particularly in view of the fact that the young man had already been earning his own living for some time. This represented significant progress compared with the time when he lay in bed for days on end and had been dependent on sickness and pension benefits.

Even though the attempt, just described, completely to liberate the choleric temperament of this person suffering from bipolar affect disorder had not led to the hoped-for result, it was possible all the same to confirm the significant realization that child-like joy in play is of the greatest significance in therapy during the manic phase. As an archetypally healthy condition it replaces the pathological and unstable state and represents in fact the spiritual home which forms the basic orientation for all further practising and expressing oneself in this regard.

In this description, the emphasis has been on revealing the methods developed in the light of this case. A consideration of relapses and other difficulties has been avoided in favour of the clearest possible overview.

The circumstance that several people with bipolar disorder were coming to me over the same period of time gave rise to an exceedingly fruitful situation, in that I was able to gain the experiences mentioned above from different points of view which mutually inspired and complemented each other, and to put the methods which I had developed to the test.

Luckily most of these patients presented less complicated conditions. I was therefore able to guide them in the way described and achieve good outcomes with them.

I would just like to mention that my isolation became a great burden to me when working with people whose illnesses brought me difficult problems. In such cases the need to present to a physician what I had discovered, and already partially put into practice, was great.

I therefore regarded as a longed-for act of providence my meeting with an eminent specialist in internal medicine, who immediately became interested in the problems which I was experiencing. His opinion and judgment, sometimes after repeated examinations of the patient at his practice, were extremely valuable to me.

Schizophrenia

In the midst of this work I was suddenly confronted with new and very challenging problems.

A woman telephoned me and said she was very poorly and would like to see me as soon as possible. There was something in her voice which disturbed me and induced me to give her the next available appointment. Luckily this was on the Friday, so that I was able to work with her over the weekend as well.

How shocked I was when she stood there before me and I looked into her eyes, which gazed at me quite madly. When she began straight away speaking of her anxieties, saying that she saw demons and heard screams, I realized the gravity of the situation.

My first thought was to have nothing to do with her, and to send her away, as I lacked the necessary insight, knowledge and experience. I also felt paralysed and could scarcely summon up the strength to withstand this demonic presence.

As the floodgates of her inner world opened ever wider and her speech became more and more confused and carried away, I began to fear that her agitated soul might be completely swallowed up by these murky, threatening forces — and then what?

I stood and walked to the window, looking for a redemptive thought. It was dusk outdoors and lights were already lit here and there. Night fell and aggravated the hopeless situation ... If only I could summon that physician or ask advice. But he was away and could not be reached then.

I turned once more to the patient. Her mad gaze fell on me and I could guess at her terrible anxiety. I shuddered and was overcome with utter helplessness and despair, which threatened to overwhelm me. The danger and a growing anxiety that I would not be able to withstand it, the responsibility which burdened me more and more, all seemed to suffocate me.

And she sat before me and stared into empty space ... The flow of her speech had run dry. A menacing silence emphasized her suffering.

Poor, tortured soul! If only I could shelter you in my deep compassion. If only I could find a beacon to shed its light on the night within you!

Then, suddenly, in this utter distress, the redemptive thought that it had been possible to find a way with depression and bipolar disorder rose up victoriously within me, filling me with a wonderful confidence and hope. I also now noticed a certain similarity between the state of loosening and being carried away in mania and the condition of this patient. I quickly decided at once to risk working with her in a similar way.

She was still staring inconsolably when I called to her and we began working, tentatively at first, then, when I was convinced she could endure it, with greater energy and determination: K K K intoned vigorously, supported by the eurythmy gesture, as we stood facing each other, speaking simultaneously. Then later on in the same way:

> Ich wehre dir den Weg,
> Ich wehre dir den Steg
>
> Defending the way,
> Defending the stage

We practised this, transformed by the imagination, until her soul was consolidated to such an extent that her gaze lost its crazy flickering.

Even though her whole condition had improved, I was unable to take responsibility for letting her return alone to her flat. I therefore offered her the ottoman in the next room. As she was still very anxious and I was concerned that she might entertain thoughts of suicide, I asked her to leave the door to the corridor open.

I lay down on the bed in my room, not to sleep, but in order to remain awake throughout the night. I had left my bedroom door open as well, so that not a sound would escape my attention.

My patient seemed calmer next morning, her gaze more normal. I worked in a similar way to the previous day with the difference that, toward the end of the session, I introduced exercises with K: Komm Kerl! (Come cur!) and so on. In this way it was possible to improve her condition to such an extent that she no longer saw or heard anything terrifying. But her whole state was so fragile that I considered it advisable for her to remain at my place for another night. Once again I stayed awake all night in the next room.

The next day, Sunday, there was further, decisive progress. After I had repeatedly carried out E and K exercises with her, her condition had became more normal, and I went on to the I, that joyful activation of self-assertion. Practising in this way, complemented by breath exercises for the first time, calmed and strengthened her soul, now released from its great distress, so that I was able to risk letting her go home.

In order to consolidate what had already been achieved and prevent a relapse into pathological clairvoyance, she began coming regularly for therapy sessions.

I then began to supplement the above exercises with trochees and dactyls while walking backwards, in the way described earlier, and with the B (done eurythmically with the legs).

I went on to work with her in a similar way to that described for stabilizing the manic state. Imitating a bull was also a great help for this patient; for she had hardly attained the capacity to stand firmly on the ground and see what is near and tangible. The compulsion to lose herself in a dissociated, floating state was countered by striving for what was clearly tangible and susceptible of earthly understanding: the bull standing in the field. This was imitated. The firm stance and connection with the earth was practised until it was possible to act freely out of this attitude.

Rolling balls was then practised to complement this work. The urge for movement which this awakened, and the direction of her attention wholly to what lay outside her, activated the joy of play from the time before puberty, unclouded by the passions. A condition of pristine health began to replace the pathological. It had to be strengthened and secured to such an extent that it could be called on at any moment until it became permanent, giving the inner support that in future would be able to regulate psychic vacillation.

The moment had come to address the great weakness in her soul, her uncertainty and diffidence. I was able to draw on the therapeutic methods I had developed for the depressive illness of the student whose case I described at the start. Like him, she had never fully entered into life, had avoided difficulties and kept clear of conflict. Since the young man had been able to acquire a remarkable inner strengthening through the warlike games which I staged, I hoped to achieve analogous results with similar (appropriate to her womanly nature) aggressive challenges.

I had not deceived myself. There soon appeared an unexpected energy and spiritual presence. Her true being began to force its way through and work its way up out of her pitiful debility.

The only disappointment for me in this positive development was that her marked lack of social contact had hardly improved. Where could the causes for this lie?

In order not to badger my patient with questions, I began to work in the following way: gently, very tenderly, I intoned an A, supported by the eurythmy gesture. She followed suit, but so hesitantly that I encouraged her to express herself with more conviction. At that she collapsed in tears.

In a later session I ventured to take up the A again, and attempted once more to release her blocked capacity to experience. However this made such a deep impact on her terrible, painful wound that she began to weep once more, loudly and bitterly, and a flood of tears stifled her voice.

I felt that the cause of the secret suffering that was gnawing away at her was beginning to struggle to the surface. What I had surmised was confirmed to me in the most shocking way: her mother had never really loved her and had therefore always foisted her off on other people. This withdrawal of love, which she had most probably had to suffer since she was a babe in arms, was the main causation of her grave illness of the soul. This is where the wall of ice was constructed which she could never have broken through by herself. Poor, poor soul!

When we took up the therapeutic speech work again, it was primarily a matter of consolidating and strengthening her churned-up, raw soul.

I chose the exercises with E and K mentioned above:

> Ich wehre dir den Weg,
> Ich wehre dir den Steg ...
> Komm, kurzer kräftiger Kerl!
>
> Defending the way,
> Defending the stage ...
> Come crooked, craftiest cur!

The result was so good that it was possible to take up once more what I had originally striven for. So we intoned A with the eurythmic gesture in the way described above; or, depending on the situation, just eurythmically or just in speech. I then went on to the hu hu hu breath exercises followed by:

> In den unermesslich weiten Räumen,
> In den endenlosen Zeiten,
> In der Menschenseele Tiefen,
> In der Welten Offenbarung:
> Suche des grossen Rätsels Lösung.

> In the vast unmeasured worldwide spaces,
> In the endless stream of time,
> In the depths of human soul-life,
> In the world's great revelations,
> Seek the unfolding of life's great mystery.

We worked line by line, in a similar way to that described at the beginning. The in-breath filled with wonder, surrendering oneself trustingly to an experience of the 'unmeasured worldwide spaces,' of the 'endless stream of time,' so that these pour into one's being, and nothing impedes or obstructs what is manifesting. Then, filled with devotion, shaping in the out-breath what has been thus received. In order to bring this way of practising into direct relation to the lack of social contact, I chose the verse for Taurus from Rudolf Steiner's Twelve Moods:

> Erhelle dich, Wesensglanz,
> Erfühle die Werdekraft,
> Verwebe den Lebensfaden
> In wesendes Weltensein,
> In sinniges Offenbaren,
> In leuchtendes Seins-Gewahren.
> O Wesensglanz, erscheine!

> Come forth, you lustre of being,
> Feel well the power of becoming,
> Enweave the thread of life
> Into being's essence of worlds,
> In thought revelation receiving,
> In radiance the essence perceiving.
> O lustre of being, appear![3]

The injunction expressed here, to 'enweave the thread of life' into being's essence of worlds, went right to the heart of the matter.

I can still see today how the thawing of her soul was reflected in her countenance as, in trusting devotion and with a good deal of breath, I let flow to her the exercise hu hu hu that we had practised in the last few sessions. Tearfully she breathed back to me what she had thus received. And the icy wall, which had guarded her inmost being for so long, began to melt.

In similar fashion to the games for agility described above, I now tried to maintain a lively, alternating intoning of the hu hu hu in a gently oscillating movement back and forth. From this point on her capacity for imitation was activated and she was able, almost without noticing it, to achieve a breakthrough into normal, natural and easy communication with another human being.

As she began visibly to blossom with this liberating activity, I experienced the rightness of it, which led me to give it plenty of time in the next few sessions. The therapy continued with exercises beginning with blown sounds:

> Sieh silberne Segel auf fliessendem Wasser
> Du zweifelst, du zürnest, du zerreissest zornig
> Zweifle nicht, zürne nicht, zerreisse nicht zornig
> Ach forsche rasch;
> Es schoss so scharf aus Schussweite
> Halt! Hebe hurtig hohe Humpen!
> Hole Heinrich hierher hohe Halme
> Weiche wehendem Winde auf Wiesenwegen

The outcome was very gratifying. It confirmed that this way of working could considerably improve the most pitiable conditions involving lack of human contact. However it was also abundantly clear that improvements of this kind would be impossible without the preparatory work described. The soul must be healthy and strong before it can make an intimate approach to another human being.

Supplementary case study

When this essay was on my desk ready for print and I had already given up my therapeutic speech work for reasons of age and ill-health, I was called on to take it up again by a woman who was suffering deeply.

She complained of terrible pains in her back, which had started years before and had since become steadily worse. Moving her limbs was so painful that she was bed-ridden. Getting up was such torture that she dreaded it. In spite of that, and at her doctor's insistence, she attempted to get on her feet from time to time and take a few steps with the help of a carer.

Because the treatment up to that point, even during a six-week hospitalization, had brought no relief, she had continually to rely on painkillers. There seemed no way out of the situation — only depression, anxiety and despair.

She begged me for help. The misery of this poor person touched me so deeply that I could not refuse.

In order to convey most clearly the struggle with her illness, what follows are the notes I made after each session.

First session, February 15

Frau S was brought to me. Her utter helplessness and the way her face became distorted by pain at the slightest attempt to move made a deep impression on me. I had not imagined it would be this extreme; I had never seen anything like it. She told me that the birth-pangs of her two 24-hour labours were nothing compared to the agony which she was suffering now. In spite of it all, her energy and determination were still perceptible. She was still marked by the extraordinary achievements.

This led me to the immediate insight that her tireless activity had been the cause of her illness. Restless activity and her constant efforts to push things through had disturbed her body's vital functions and probably overwhelmed them on occasion, which had eventually led to cramps and complete disability.

For this reason I directed my activity to the passive pole of behaviour, quite indirectly and approaching the matter very obliquely: we would have to make space, learn to conduct ourselves so that the life of our organism was not strained or damaged. We would have to acquire passivity in the sense of allowing things to happen, not as floppiness but as a willingness to allow oneself to be acted upon.

In this way we liberate the life pole of existence. It can find its way back to the life processes which hold sway in it and which are filled with and guided by lofty wisdom.

We began to work toward this goal by intoning and forming eurythmically A O U. This was able to shine the first glimmer of light into her darkness. She left after the session in the hope that the aim of her future quest might lie in what I had offered.

With great difficulty she was helped out of the house and into a car to be taken home.

Second session, February 18

Frau S's son drove her over. She was in a very bad state, quite crushed and in a very deep depression.

'It was all so terrible,' she sighed. 'My husband telephoned his brother during my first session with you. His brother is friendly with the medical director of a clinic in Berne, and they ended up discussing my condition. The doctor then advised that, in order that at last something rational and responsible may be undertaken, I should be admitted to his department, examined thoroughly and treated. In my utter weakness and helplessness, I submitted to their will. I will now go through with all of this and get in touch with you afterwards,' she told me.

Concerned not to show my disappointment, I took up again what we had begun to establish in the first session (intoning and forming eurythmically A O U). In this way I was able to consolidate and calm down her distraught state again.

Her son then arrived to collect her in his car. He at once began a very good and fruitful conversation. He felt that my methods should first be given an opportunity to show their potential for healing, before trying other approaches. And that is how it continued.

Third session, February 21

Frau S again complained of terrible pains and of the impact of her many painkillers. (She forgets everything and feels demoralized and depressed.) To my surprise, however, she is determined to continue working with me. The family too is now committed to it, thanks to the firm conviction of her son who vociferously and very insistently put forward the view that it is absolutely essential for this treatment, which he now believes in since his conversation with me, to be given a chance.

In spite of this gratifying outcome, it was difficult getting the work going again. In a similar way to the previous two sessions, I was aiming toward a condition where she would become sufficiently passive, allowing things to happen. From a different starting point to that in the first session, I tried to give Frau S to understand that we must sometimes allow the realm of the invisible to work on our life, guiding it, and not interrupt this subtle working with our own actions.

In order to help her experience this, I lifted her arms, which had been hanging down. She immediately helped in this. It took a great effort on her part before she was able to let me lift her arms without her help. But when she succeeded, her pains disappeared for a moment. This wonderful discovery confirmed that we were on the right path. We were now fully committed to begin a reverent standing back to give space to the mysterious realm of our existence. Thus on several occasions she succeeded in letting me lift her limply hanging arms without her assistance. The pains disappeared on each occasion.

Then, to test this deeply moving event, she moved her arms in the previous way and the pains returned at once. So we tentatively tried a few more times what we had found to work, and always had the same, almost inexplicable, pain-free outcome.

Fourth session, February 24

I resumed the lifting of her passive arms which in the previous session had worked successfully. This was now going so well that I could venture to approach her still terribly painful back. She now had to apply in this area what she had managed in allowing her arms to be lifted: without giving the slightest resistance or help she had to give herself over to my attempt very gently and slightly to bend her back and straighten it up again. Lo and behold — it worked! The pains disappeared for a moment. Frau S had grasped the essence, and it only remained to make it her own through diligent practice.

She soon learned, when bending and straightening her back, to simply 'let it happen' even without my help. And each time her pains disappeared for a moment.

We experienced this as a true miracle, in face of which our thinking and conventional knowledge had to retreat with reverence. Our experience alone was able to convince us and more and more decidedly became our guiding star.

Fifth session, March 3
Frau S was unable to carry on with what we had achieved in the previous session. So we built up again and practised what had been introduced then.

Sixth session, March 6
As Frau S is still too much bound up in her awareness of her painful back, I began to refocus her consciousness into intensive playful movement of fingers and hands, toes and feet.

A completely limp arm is guided through the space; the other hand grasps it and moves it in circling, gently swinging movements rhythmically up and down, back and forth. This game was a great help.

I support Frau S under one arm and guide her, as smoothly as possible, toward a goal which she has clearly in view, so that it is as if she were carried along by me.

In all these exercises, the part of her body which needed moving was as it were taken hold of and guided from without. The outcome was amazing: the stiffness was gone and her body was pain-free.

This condition was maintained until a movement was inadvertently carried out in the old way.

Seventh session, March 9
Frau S arrived in a much improved condition. We went through again what we had worked on in the previous session.

Then we turned our attention once more to the idea of being led from outside ourselves. We looked at how we may be helped if we are willing to realize that we are in need of help, and learn to adopt an attitude of devotion.

Eighth session, March 12
For the first time Frau S got out of her husband's car without a stick.

We practised my taking hold of her limply hanging arms and moving them upward, which she permitted without her own participation; bending and straightening her back, as described above; and walking toward a goal — I am led, my body is drawn forward.

At the end of the session Frau S was free of pain. This miracle was wrought by her allowing it to happen, letting herself be guided without resistance.

Ninth session, March 16
Frau S arrived in a good state. The effects of the previous session had been very good. We therefore worked in the same way again.

Tenth session, March 19
Frau S arrived in a bad way. She had been working too intensely, and felt it in her back again. However the pains had not returned again; instead she felt an unpleasant tingling.

So we once more practised my holding and moving her loosely hanging arms upward and bending and straightening her back.

Eleventh session, March 24
Frau S arrived in a good state. In the last few sessions she has made some fine progress in allowing herself to be acted upon.

To complement that, attention to the realm of the invisible was emphasized. This realm of life, brimming with events replete with wisdom, should not be disturbed by hectic hustle and bustle or an aggressively impetuous will. Her new deep insight showed her that what is needed here is reverent restraint, which leads directly to the attitude of soul expressed through allowing oneself to be acted on.

Twelfth session, March 30
The day after the previous session, Frau S was still completely free of pain. She cooked lunch again for the first time. As the tingling in her back had begun again after this exertion, I worked in the same way as on March 12: taking hold of her limply hanging arms and moving them upward; bending and straightening her back; and walking toward a goal — I am led, my body is drawn forward.

Thirteenth session, April 6
Frau S has been working too hard and has had a relapse, and was unable to carry through what we worked on in the previous session.

I therefore felt it necessary to take up again what we had been working on in the previous sessions: we concentrated on raising her limply hanging arms and bending and straightening her back. Particular attention was paid to allowing it to happen and to the feeling in the soul of being acted upon from without. This helped so much that Frau S was free of pain again by the end of the session.

Fourteenth session, April 27
Frau S arrived in a good state and without her stick. She managed the Easter holidays in spite of all the strain and stress.

As she still gets stiff sometimes when walking, I began our work by having her start from a completely relaxed posture, really floppy, and then shuffle forward with slightly bent knees. This worked really well as a variation.

We then worked again on bending and straightening her back: we are aided; we let our back bend; we let it be straightened once more. This dispelled the last remaining tingling.

After this had been repeated several times with the same satisfactory results, the next step toward normalizing the process of movement could be ventured upon. We began very gently to let our will, filled with guiding power, flow into the unfolding process which had been entrusted to the organism and grew from it.

In this way we built up anew the processes of movement in our limbs and our body, in a way akin to the instinctual behaviour impressed into us by nature, which has become lost.

Fifteenth session, May 4
Frau S came on foot from the station, which represented great progress. The work in the previous session had had a really good effect. This showed clearly that our goal was attainable, and that all that remained was to work at what had been discovered until the lost, instinctive behaviour was wholly replaced by what could be achieved by conscious activity. I then repeated what we had worked on in the previous session.

Sixteenth session, May 18
Frau S arrived in a good state. She is really getting on amazingly well now: she is cooking again and doing various bits of housework and gardening once more. She has also gone out for a meal with her husband, which she had not managed for a long, long time.

She is striving to live a normal, healthy life, cares for her appearance and looks young and pretty.

As the work in the previous two sessions had had such positive results, we continued to work in a similar way.

Seventeenth session, May 25

Frau S was once more in a good state when she came. She says that it is still not always possible for her to reach this good state. She still needs my help, particularly when working on consciously carried-out movement processes. We therefore practised in the same way as in the previous sessions.

The fact that help from the divine worlds flows towards us in all that we undertake has once more become a deep experience for her. We are guided and helped when we place ourselves in the right way into the world.

Eighteenth session, June 1

Frau S was in a good way when she arrived. As the previous sessions had brought good results, I repeated what we had worked on in them.

Nineteenth session, June 9

Frau S was in a very good state when she came. She had consulted her physician for the first time in many weeks, and he was amazed at her recovery. He told her that the whole musculature of her back, which at the time of her previous examination had still been very hard, had softened again and was completely normal. This assessment, and his judgment that the cure was an extraordinary achievement, I found very valuable, as they confirmed that both my understanding of the illness and what we undertook as therapy had been right.

Frau S then told me that she had now got hold of the conscious way of moving which we had worked on in our sessions: 'For instance, when I want to get up from a chair, I don't just go at it any old how, like I used to, but I contain myself and allow the feeling of being determined from outside to arise in me. At the same time I feel that I make room for a wonderfully wise event, as if my body is being prepared to take up the impulse for movement, which I have deliberately activated, and carry it out. This gives me a really agreeable feeling. Then when I carry out the movement, I experience it as an utterly healthy undertaking, which is now able completely consciously to bring about the paradisal state of an instinctive happening, as things were before my illness.'

When she had finished this excellent description of the process she had been through, we proceeded to some of the exercises mentioned already which were appropriate to the current situation.

Twentieth session, June 23

Frau S arrived in a very good, completely normal state. She has managed to make her own what we have worked on over this whole period in conversations and practical exercises.

Her movements are now completely pain-free and appear fluent and beautiful. As she is immediately aware of wrong movements as they occur, and can correct them, it would now be right to bring our work to a conclusion.

The whole experience had made a deep impression on us both; it was exhilarating and beautiful, a real grace.

It will be apparent from the therapeutic speech methods which have been described that they are not universally applicable. In that they require intimate, intensive and consistent work on oneself, they will be of real help to those who long for an inner direction, strengthening and harmonization in their lives.

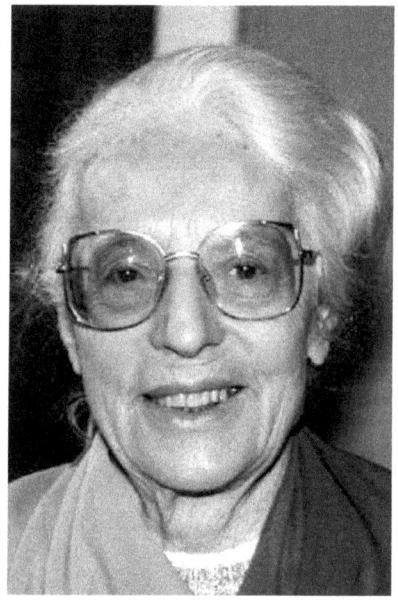

Dora Gutbrod, March 18, 1905 – June 25, 1989

Dora Gutbrod

Autobiography

Dora Gutbrod was born on March 18, 1905, as second of three children of a happy Stuttgart family. Her father, a physician, was gifted artistically, fond of learning, and enjoyed life to the full. Her mother worked as an editor at a prominent Stuttgart publisher, and was interested in the spiritual life.

There was much music in the family. Her brother, who was three years older, subsequently trained as an opera singer. Dora became a speech artist and actress, her younger brother Rolf an architect. The family home stood at the heart of a large family: her father's four brothers, who were scattered around the world, regarded it as their focal point; Dora's grandmother lived there until she was in her hundredth year.

Dora's mother did not agree with the educational methods of that time, and had engaged a private tutor called Adam Braun for Dora's elder brother and the similarly-aged son of a friend. This tutor introduced her to anthroposophy and to Rudolf Steiner. She became a member of the Anthroposophical Society in 1916.

Dora Gutbrod's long relationship with Günther Sponholz and her deep friendship with Madeleine van Deventer, the medical director of the Ita Wegman Clinic, were decisive for her destiny. When her stage career came to an end, she began collaborating energetically with doctors and teachers. In her last years, Dora was often asked by young people to tell them about her life. At the same time she wrote this account of her life, with which we are now able to continue in her own words.

Ursula Ostermai

In Autumn 1919 the Waldorf School was founded by Rudolf Steiner and Emil Molt. The opening ceremony took place in the City Park. First some of the children showed the poem 'The Frogs' by Lethe in eurythmy — I was thrilled — then Rudolf Steiner came and gave a talk to the teachers, parents and children. My heart went out to him, and it was probably one of the most significant moments in my life up to then.

In spite of the fact that Rudolf Steiner spoke for at least an hour or more, I was deeply impressed by his appearance and the power of his voice, which was filled with warmth — though of course I cannot recall what he said. We were deeply moved by the powerful and intense way he spoke to us children; the thought stirred in me that I would like to study and get to know this way of speaking. How this might come about was a complete mystery to me.

In the afternoon, the 250 children went to the Uhlandshöhe [where the school had its site], and each teacher called their class together. I entered Class 8 — and never regretted it! My brother Rolf joined Class 3. We Class 8 pupils went up to Dr Treichler, later our French teacher, and he raced with us across the playground. I had never come across a teacher who did such a thing.

Herr Molt stood on the steps holding a huge laundry basket, from which he gave us a small packet of chocolate and biscuits to send us on our way. This was a miracle in the year 1919, as there was widespread poverty after the war, and most children had never had any chocolate.

The beginning of school! You may be aware that our school was housed in a restaurant and café. Our classroom did not have any benches. We sat on garden chairs with our exercise books on our laps; I do not recall how long this continued.

Our teachers were Walter Johannes Stein, Karl Stockmeyer, later Erich Schwebsch, Karl Schubert, Paul Baumann for music, and Elisabeth Baumann, our revered eurythmy teacher. When Rudolf Steiner visited the school and walked across the playground in break time, the little ones rushed up to him, each one wanting to shake his hand, and the call of 'Good morning, Dr Steiner!' filled the air. We older ones stood at a seemly distance while he gave one hand to the little ones and waved to us with the other!

My impression was that all the teachers were radiantly happy that they could be Waldorf teachers. Rudolf Steiner frequently visited the school then and came into lessons as well. It was probably in Class 10 that Rudolf Steiner asked us about the soul forces. We gave the stupidest answers and noticed that Rudolf Steiner was very disappointed in us. Then our teacher, Walter Johannes Stein, went to stand behind Rudolf Steiner and held up three fingers. We all realized at once what the answer was and I thought to myself that, as Rudolf Steiner was clairvoyant, he must have noticed Dr Stein holding up three fingers.

One great difficulty was that half of us came from more advanced schools, whereas the children of the workers at the Waldorf Astoria factory were from elementary schools; alas, alas, half the class was bored, even though the teachers tried their best to be even-handed. After I left the school in 1922, I always remembered the way Rudolf Steiner stood before us, and always concluded his address with the words, 'Children, do you love your teachers?' Since being permitted to participate in the Speech and Drama Course at the age of 19, I have never forgotten his gestures.

The question of my profession now came up. I was attracted to eurythmy, but speech formation fascinated me even more. It was not so much that it particularly appealed to me, more that I was disappointed by what I heard from friends at drama schools. My father, who was a physician, suffered from a serious heart condition, and we were permitted to come to his bedroom in the evening and listen to Schiller's ballads. In August 1924 I saw an announcement in the Goetheanum for the Speech and Drama Course. This electrified me and I besieged Dr Kühn and his wife with my requests to allow me to take part in this course. At that time, I was working as an au pair in the Kühn household.

As Frau Dr Steiner was coming to Stuttgart with the eurythmists for a performance, I went to the show and applied for an interview with her. There was a long queue of people waiting to see her, and I was chosen to go in first.

She was sitting in a large room. When I gave her a deep curtsey on entering the room, she said kindly, 'Do come a little closer.' I held her in too great esteem to do so.

She asked, 'What is your purpose in coming to see me?' then asked me to recite something for her.

Unfortunately I was unable to think of anything. 'You could also do an exercise,' she said. In a loud voice, I spoke the exercise Dass er dir log ...

'You do not have to speak it so loudly!'

I then asked her if I might take part in the Speech and Drama Course. She asked my age.

'Nineteen.'

'I shall talk the matter over with Rudolf Steiner.'

Two weeks later I received my invitation signed by Rudolf Steiner.

During the Speech and Drama Course I was a guest of the Kühns, and slept on a straw mattress at the foot of Mrs Kühn's bed.

After the course, I returned to Köngen, where I remained until March 10, 1925. My application of March 15, 1925 to Marie Steiner, asking to participate in her work with the actors, was turned down, with a suggestion that I enter the Eurythmy School in Stuttgart. That was the last thing I wanted to do!

On March 30 we heard of Rudolf Steiner's death. None of us was able to grasp it, nor did we want to.

On April 20 I received a letter from Dornach. Frau Dr Steiner was organizing a speech course, led by Herr Froböse. I was enthusiastic about this; it was now a matter of persuading my father to give me permission and to provide the wherewithal for me to go to Dornach. He agreed that I might stay there for three months. I had had my twentieth birthday in March.

The course took place in Hansi House, where Dr and Frau Steiner had lived.

After the course had been running for six weeks, Marie Steiner came in one day, and said to Herr Froböse, 'Just carry on with your lesson.' On Marie Steiner's appearance my knees turned to jelly. When it came to my turn, I decided to tell a white lie, and declared that I was unable to speak as I was hoarse.

After another six weeks I repeated the same trick. After the lesson, Frau Dr Steiner had me come out to her and said, 'Dr Steiner prescribed me a remedy against hoarseness,' and described it very exactly. 'You can gargle with it and drink it too.' With the last of my money I purchased the raspberry juice that I needed for it.

After I had been taking part in Herr Froböse's course for about four months, a speech formation artist asked me to read for eurythmy, as she herself had been admitted into Mrs Steiner's lessons. Boldly I replied that I would be glad to try it.

On the Tuesday afternoon Marie Steiner came into the eurythmy rehearsal, asked to be shown what they were practising, then drew up the programme for the following Sunday. I read a poem for one of the eurythmists. All Marie Steiner said was, 'No, that is not yet ready; as for what the young lady was reading, I couldn't understand a single word.'

I thought to myself that this was not exactly a good beginning! In the course of the rehearsal we came to the poem 'Urtrieb' by Fercher von Steinwand. Frau Dr Steiner had already rejected six actors, and declared, 'If no-one can read it we shall have to leave it out.' The leading eurythmist, Tatiana Kisselev, pointed to me and said, 'She has also been reading.'

'Has she?' said Marie Steiner. 'As far as I am concerned, she can have a try.'

I made my trembling way up to the stage and began, expecting an interruption at any moment. But none came!

The poem was two pages long. After I had finished, Marie Steiner stood up, came over to me in her laboured way, and said, 'You will read this for the eurythmy performance on Sunday.'

She took my book and marked the places where I should pause to take a breath.

In the following rehearsal, Marie Steiner said, 'The young girl should come to my rehearsal.'

Shortly afterward I was sitting in on the rehearsals with my head burning. It was absolutely clear to me that this was what I wanted to learn! It did not occur to me that it would turn out to be so hard.

It should be emphasized that after Rudolf Steiner's death Marie Steiner took on the heavy task of producing the Mystery Plays for the second Goetheanum, which was yet to be built, as well as preparing major eurythmy performances and speech choruses with the available actors. The hard work had begun.

In December 1925, we began work on the Temple Scene from The Portal of Initiation for Rudolf Steiner's anniversary on February 27, 1926. I was given the role of Luna, one of the soul forces, which I then kept for the next fourteen years. Erna Grund had the part of Astrid and, to begin with, Hertha Louise Zuelzer that of Philia.

If Marie Steiner came to the rehearsal at 11.15, it went on till 2.30 or 3 o'clock, sometimes till 3.30 pm! Well, what was her way of working like? She gave out the parts and the rehearsal began. Tirelessly she spoke all the lines for us to repeat. After a week Frau Dr Steiner had worked on perhaps one scene. The following week and the one after, it was the same scene. Everyone was expected to attend all the rehearsals, regardless of whether they were in the scene or not. We began to realize that we had no idea how a sentence could be shaped in a living way, or what was involved in speaking on the breath, bringing the sounds to life, or speaking in a way that was not intellectual.

Marie Steiner's great task was to awaken in us an understanding of how the works of Rudolf Steiner, Goethe, Schiller, Nietzsche, Hebbel and Morgenstern should be spoken. She was also able to inspire us with the grandeur of the German language.

The eurythmy rehearsals: when it had reached 3.00 pm and the third part had not even been started on, our first violin, Max Schuurman, would often come with his instrument under his arm, wait till there was a short break, and say that the musicians were unable to stay 'for a little night music.' Marie Steiner would say with a sigh, Oh well then, you can play all the music pieces through one after the other; after that I have to continue working with the speakers.'

If one had to speak in the third part, Marie Steiner was very tired after four hours of strenuous rehearsal, and the atmosphere could become tense. One often did a colleague an injustice by thinking to oneself, 'Won't he ever get it right?' Then it was one's own turn, and one was even worse ...

However, the chorus rehearsals took the biscuit! Standing on the same spot for hour after hour! By two o'clock in the afternoon Marie Steiner's patience was exhausted. She would shout, 'You're not trying hard enough; your commitment is not strong enough; there's no fire!' And the ultimate threat, 'One at a time, please —'

Woe betide you, if Marie Steiner decided to change a programme: the first item came third, the third first; we called that the 'grandfather', and knew it would go on for an eternity.

September 1928! The opening of the second Goetheanum. Two thousand members came. Everything had to be shown twice. From June onwards, the actors were in the Goetheanum every evening from 7.30 onward. On the first night, the rehearsal ended at 3.30 in the morning!

Jan Stuten had suggested an orchestra pit which could be raised and lowered. There was a gaping hole in front of the stage, with a low railing round it, so that Marie Steiner would not fall down it (it was her first time in the hall). There were neither seats nor lighting; we were surrounded by deepest night. We were supposed to try and find the best acoustics, so we climbed up onto the gallery. It then took us another half-hour to reach the auditorium once more. At two in the morning Mare Steiner said, 'Whoever is tired may go; I am still going to read "The Nature and Origin of the Arts".' (She was going to read this at the opening ceremony.) Two of the Mystery Plays had been prepared.

Only later, in 1932, was the first part of Faust ready. Erna Grund excelled in a harrowing performance as Gretchen, Hendewerk played Faust and Bevan Redlich was Mephisto.

All I remember is how during the applause which did not seem as if it would ever end Marie Steiner stood up in tears and said something along the lines of, 'It was not all quite how I would have liked it!'

What was the effect of the speech impulse which fired Marie Steiner? What was its significance? What did her pupils experience over and again when they succeeded in climbing a few steps only to plunge once more into the yawning chasm, from which they struggled to extract themselves?

Out of these three years of work between 1925 and 1928, the speech chorus came about. It both fulfilled and inspired us; between 1928 and 1935 it brought us considerable recognition. During that time the speech chorus went on tour every autumn for four to six weeks.

In Berlin, our performances were often sold out far in advance. A while ago I read the reviews: Berlin, Breslau, Hamburg, and so forth. I had almost forgotten what a runaway success the chorus was! After that our performances in Germany were banned: in 1935 the Anthroposophical Society in Germany was outlawed.

Why is speech formation initially so alienating for many people? It is because we are no longer aware that the sounds have their origin in the cosmos: the vowels are assigned to the planets, the consonants to the zodiac.

We practised Christian Morgenstern's poem for Rudolf Steiner:

ER SPRACH ...

Er sprach. Und wie er sprach, erschien in ihm
der Tierkreis, Cherubim und Seraphim,
der Sonnenstern, der Wandel der Planeten
von Ort zu Ort.
Das alles sprang hervor bei seinem Laut,
ward blitzschnell, wie ein Weltentraum, erschaut,
der ganze Himmel schien herabgebeten
bei seinem Wort.

He spoke. And, as he spoke, appeared in him
the zodiac, cherubim and seraphim,
the starry sun, the journey of the planets
from place to place.
It all sprang forth when his voice sounded,
was glimpsed in a flash, a cosmic dream,
the whole of heaven appeared invited down to us
upon his word.

Marie Steiner said, 'The sounds are messengers of the gods, you must redeem them through your speaking!' Yes, Morgenstern certainly showed us this in his poem, but the path! How good it was that the chorus was able to exist and that the fire of 24 young people blazed up as one. Admittedly chorus speaking calls for renunciation, but we dearly wished to reach beyond ourselves in order to meet again on a higher plane.

Marie Steiner cried, 'Place your breath at the disposal of the sounds so that they may become free to resound in the roundelay of the spheres!' Could there have been a nobler task? In the beginning, none of us guessed how hard this was; but if we managed to take hold of the slightest part of it, none of us could ever let go again. Each of us was impelled to continue on the path. Each individual had to seek and strive with their best effort, but also to listen in humility when told that they had not succeeded. Listen to yourself! Don't just sound beautiful!

There were rehearsals where it became clear what it meant 'to guide light into the tone, open up the concept, penetrate into the depths, go through the portal of turning.'

'Yes,' Marie Steiner would say, 'that is the music of the future; you have a whole scale of tones in your soul — carry us along with you to experience the poem or the character. Burst your bounds and expand!'

There were moments when this became our own experience. You couldn't hold on to anything any more; instead there was a new wakefulness, which had not been there before; this always had to be sought anew through the force of our I. We can only speak when the I is stirred to activity by the power of the spirit.

The chorus practised the words given by Rudolf Steiner for the coloured glass windows of the Goetheanum.

Red window: Ich schaue ... (I behold)

Frau Dr Steiner: 'Go through the Sch into the Au and release it in the E. Be inspired by the eurythmic Sch, then gently into the sun-sound Au and let it die away in the E.'

Es offenbart ... (It reveals)

Suddenly one felt how the two Fs open up, then the sobering admonition came, 'Please let us not have a beard at the end, fill the A with light!'

Es hat geoffenbart ... (It has revealed)

'The past, it has taken place, irrevocable.'

Mauve window: So wird er fromm ... (Thus he becomes pious)

'Feel the double M! Speak diaphanously!'

Die Welt weht Frommsein ... (The world wafts piety)

'Unless you experience the W both times, you cannot shape!'

Die Frommheit wirkt ... (Piety is working)

'Everything is consolidated through the K. Make for the wirkt and come down to earth with the K.'

In recollection this rehearsal appears as a path of catharsis.

From the rehearsals of the Easter choruses from Faust Part I:

> Faust: Welch tiefes Summen, welch ein heller Ton
> Zieht mit Gewalt das Glas von meinem Munde?

> What deep humming, what bright tone
> Violently tears the glass from my lips?

After the sung chorus came the speech chorus from behind thick curtains:

Freude dem Sterblichen ... (Joy to the mortal one)

'No, no,' resounded from the auditorium, 'I can't hear a word.' After we had tried our uttermost for about half an hour, and Marie Steiner had become more and more impatient, she said, 'Please come forward into the auditorium!' Frau Dr Steiner could probably hear that we were doing our best; she spoke the text sublimely, but the mass of curtains behind which the chorus was standing, and through which it was meant to resound, robbed it time and again of the angelic tone that was striven for.

Then the penitents. 'Please let us feel the tears, it has to be spoken downward.' The penitents were spoken by five women; hardly had the first line sounded forth, when there was a mighty tempest: sentimentality utterly incensed Marie Steiner. Then the chorus of disciples rang out, and the women were relieved that the men too were insufficiently celestial. Then came the climax:

    Christ ist erstanden ... (Christ has arisen)

The back wall of the set was removed, the great chorus of angels became visible — then all the stagehands rushed in so that they could experience what it meant 'to rise above oneself, release the tone and still speak with all one's power.'

Sometimes it came about that silence came over the auditorium for minutes on end. We realized then that it was not enough that the Dornach stage had a good Faust, or a very dramatic Mephisto; everyone was called on to give of their best — and this was required of us in every rehearsal. Once, when one of the actors said, 'I'm just going through the motions,' it was all we could do to prevent Marie Steiner from walking out.

There was work on lyrical poetry with individual speakers. From 'Dem Schmerz sein Recht' by Friedrich Hebbel.

    Unergründlicher Schmerz!
    Knirscht ich in vorigen Stunden:
    Jetzt, mit noch blutenden Wunden,
    Segnet und preist dich mein Herz.

    Alles Leben ist Raub;
    Funken, die Sonnen entstammen,
    Lodern, das All zu durchfallen,
    Da verschluckt sie der Staub.
    Nun ein heiliger Krieg!
    Höchste und tiefste Gewalten
    Drängen in allen Gestalten!
    Trotze, so bleibt dir der Sieg ...

    Endless agony!
    I grind my teeth in the wee small hours:
    Now, with still bleeding wounds,
    My heart blesses and glorifies you.

    All life is robbery;
    Sparks, stemming from stars,

Blaze, to put the cosmos to shame,
The dust swallows them up.
Now for holy war!
Highest and deepest powers
Press forward into all forms!
Defy them, and you'll be victorious ...

Frau Dr Steiner: 'Please, not so physical! Don't press! Feel your bone marrow!' I understood this to mean: 'You must penetrate through the hard bone to the malleable marrow, then you can portray pain convincingly.'

Marie Steiner found words of the highest praise for the poet Hebbel: 'He penetrates to the last mysteries; all you have to do is enter deeply enough.'

Es grüsst dich wohl ein Augenblick,
Der ist so überschwellend voll,
Als ob er dich mit seligem Glück
Für alle Zukunft tränken soll.
Du aber wehrst, eh du's vermeinst,
Ihn scheu und zitternd selber ab,
Und jene Träne, die du weinst,
Gibt ihm den Glanz, doch auch das Grab.
Uns dünkt die Freude Altar-Wein,
Am Heiligsten ein sündiger Raub:
Zieht Gottes Hauch durch unser Sein,
So fühlen wir uns doppelt Staub.

A moment greets you,
Full to overflowing,
As if it might water you
With bliss and joy forever.
But you reject it before you know it,
Shy and shaking,
And the tears you weep
Give it a gleam and also the grave.
Joy seems like sacramental wine,
Sinfully stolen from the Holiest:
When God's breath blows through our being,
We feel ourselves doubly as dust.

A battle with one's own feelings had to be fought in this poem. Marie Steiner: 'Hebbel is a poet of thoughts. As you speak the first line, make it bright; go quickly through the next one, and experience how Hebbel finds the only words that can express the poem. Now try to objectify it through the intensity of the consonants. Release the words in the breath. That is the key to objectivity.'

Marie Steiner's work with individual actors on stage did not consist of stage directions or attitudes one had to strike; it was work on the word, the sentence, the experience of the sound. This showed us how work with individuals enabled the whole group to learn and how we were growing together into a community.

About the work on the Mystery Plays. In 1929 (I had been in Dornach for four years) it had been very cold for several weeks already, and these external conditions obliged me to spend a few weeks in Stuttgart with my parents. I received an icy welcome on my return.

We were practising Scene 2 of The Guardian of the Threshold in the joinery. The soul forces at the end of the scene were treated harshly. My part was Luna. The conclusion of her speech went thus: 'And traces are followed by souls that are trying to search out those portals which gods have shut fast to will that errs.' Frau Dr Steiner was not happy: I just could not get the form of the sentence out. She cried, 'Go across the stage like an English setter, with your nose as close as possible to the ground, and try to make what you have to say sound convincing!'

As my colleagues roared with laughter I went about five times round the big stage in a circle, in the prescribed posture. At last I got the sentence right. Marie Steiner said, 'That's what happens when one stays in Stuttgart for so long making tutus!'

In The Guardian of the Threshold Günther Sponholz had to speak Ahriman's long piece in Scene 8. They went at it hammer and tongs for about an hour. Frau Doktor groaned, 'I'm going to shatter on this rock,' and cried, 'Sponholz, stop squawking like a Prussian lieutenant!'

That hit the mark (Sponholz had wanted to make a career as an officer in the military). I sat down near Marie Steiner, as it was sometimes possible to avert a disaster. Suddenly she called out happily, 'Do you hear? He has broken through and managed to get into his sentences.'

Bliss all round. We did not suffer only from our own inability; we also shared the suffering of our colleagues when they were unable to get to the heart of the matter.

At a rehearsal for Albert Steffen's Antichrist my colleague Gerhardt Marwitz was playing the priest. He approached me, sobbing, and said,

'Dora, I can't say, "Take the bread." Imagine that, I am unable to speak three words!'

We practised together at length, so that it was a little bit better by the next rehearsal; by no means good, but the spectre of dismissal had been banished. Dismissal meant that the victim could be sidelined for six months and only able to learn by listening.

In rehearsals for Adonis, a play by Albert Steffen the character of the sister in this play was my first leading role. It contained the sentence (one among many similar ones!): 'The daughters of Jerusalem are surely the most wonderful flower of their race, for the mother of God was born of them.' This sentence brought me close to despair.

What did Marie Steiner demand of the speakers? Certainly not an intellectual approach, but rather that they dive down into the stream of speech: 'When you speak the first line, all the rest must already be alive within you.' Through the constant repetition and practice, one gained access to one's breath and the sounds. One no longer had the security of one's understanding, but was carried beyond oneself into a newly created world.

We had to repeat things hundreds of times and exclude all our personal feelings. When Marie Steiner spoke something for us to repeat, it all seemed so simple and obvious. But woe betide you when you had to try it yourself. 'Let go, immerse yourself in the grandeur of this sentence.' One could get an inkling of what it meant to let something rise above the personal: 'Speak from the lips, release the sounds.'

At the end of the play, the sister falls into the lake, is saved by her brother and carried onto the stage, apparently dead. She comes to and describes what she experienced at the moment of death. Marie Steiner was sitting on the stage beside me, I was lying on the ground and had to say countless times, 'Yes, yes, I breathed deeply, so deeply; breathed my whole life in again,' until at last it was free of the body and rang true. What joy, when it was right at last.

Then the sister had to describe an experience of the etheric Christ. I had to speak it all after Marie Steiner, word for word; and then repeat it all the following day, always searching for the shape and formation of the sentences. Three or four hours went by in a flash for Frau Doktor and those she was working with. The other actors had to listen; in this way everyone was able to learn. Granted, one was at the limit of one's capabilities, but there were sudden flashes of insight which opened up a different world, and the actor was taken hold of by the irresistible movement.

In December 1947 — by which time Frau Dr Steiner was living in Beatenberg — I was asked whether I would like to work on Goethe's

Iphigenia. At the beginning of January 1948, the group involved in the first act set off for Beatenberg, where we spent a week working on the act. It was distressing to see how Marie Steiner had become so frail. She carried a green umbrella to shield her weakened eyes against the light. After we had greeted each other, she said, 'Now, Dora, I will only be able to give you an indication of how you should speak.'

However, her elemental power returned when she spoke the lines for us, thank God.

As far as I recall, we practised for two to three hours every morning and afternoon. Of course, Marie Steiner was exhausted after that, but her enthusiasm for this magnificent play was so great that she quite forgot herself and put body and soul into it in the usual way. The actors went to Beatenberg three times; in June only Hendewerk (Orestes) and I went, in order to speak the third act for Marie Steiner. She said, 'Very beautiful!' to which I replied, 'But Frau Doktor, I don't want to be beautiful, I want to be true!' This gladdened her and she took up the suggestion; we began all over again from the beginning. It was a strenuous but wonderful time; then we had to put all our efforts into practice.

Marie Steiner died in December 1948.

2

Therapeutic Speech and Rudolf Steiner

A Therapeutic Exercise:
An Angegebenes sieh innig hin

BARBARA DENJEAN-VON STRYCK
AND RALF UNTERBUSCH

For decades the so-called thyroid or goitre exercise has been passed on by speech formation teachers in person, usually in hand-written form, and has been worked on by groups of colleagues. Although it has frequently been applied successfully in therapeutic speech work, it has never before been published. It is one of the few therapeutic speech exercises by Rudolf Steiner for an indication beyond the speech organs in their narrow sense. There exists a typewritten sheet of paper in the archive of the Executors of Rudolf Steiner's Estate in Dornach.[1] Its author is unknown. There is a handwritten note at the top of the paper: 'for Hermann Ranzenberger'. The contents are as follows.

> Given by Dr Rudolf Steiner
> The following is to be used as a speech exercise for goitre, aloud and accentuated:
> > An Angegebenes sieh innig hin.
> > Wiege Wagnis wenig wegen Wogenwind.
> > Bete bittend und tue die Tat.
> > Gib biegend die Gabe ab.
> > Kein Nickel lasse sich auch im Kasten kleben.
> > Wenn wüstes Wasserstauen wenig wohl winkt wird winzig.
> > Errette redend den netten Retter redender Erdenrede.
> When the same consonant finishes one word and begins the next, it is important that they be spoken as distinctly separate sounds: Kein Nickel lasse, and so on. If possible the exercise should be spoken several times daily.

Apart from this one should observe one's disposition, for instance whether one soon leaves off doing something which one has undertaken to do and which needs to be carried out regularly over a longish period; however it should not be something which one does in response to external authority, but rather something one has decided on oneself. It is very good to keep at it and not leave off.

Then one should wean oneself of a certain indifference which one might experience toward some things which could actually concern one.

What is meant is not, for instance, considering something is beneath one, but rather complacency, lack of interest, perhaps even apathy.

Closer study of this exercise reveals the multifaceted and differentiated way in which Rudolf Steiner applies speech as a remedy, out of a spiritual understanding of the human being, and incorporates it through the breath into the blood and metabolism. In order to grasp the therapeutic implications of this, let us look at the thyroid gland and its pathology.

The thyroid gland

The position of the thyroid gland can alert the attentive observer to the essential tasks of this small organ. It lies directly below the larynx, enveloping, from the front, the windpipe and the bottom part of the larynx. With a paired form, shaped like a butterfly, it suggests a small lung in the upper part of the airy organization.

It informs the whole lower human being with the astralizing forces of the air. Sensitively it regulates the relation of the organization of the nerves and senses to the metabolism. Its direct connection with the autonomic nervous system becomes very clear when one visualizes the polar opposite nature of pathological deviations of the thyroid function.

If the thyroid is working too strongly, producing too much hormonal substance, then all the symptoms of an excessive activity of the sympathetic nervous system appear. Where there is insufficient hormonal production the effect can be observed in the parasympathetic nervous system.

The first case leads to overexcited wakefulness; in the second, fatigue, listlessness and exhaustion predominate. However, hyperactivity and hypoactivity of the thyroid can go over into each other. In both cases the illness can lead to the forming of goitre, which itself can arise during normal hormone production.

Overactive thyroid	Underactive thyroid
too much day consciousness	too much night consciousness
enhanced metabolism	reduced metabolism
tendency to higher temperature	lower bodily temperature
quicker pulse, possibly arrhythmic	slower, thready pulse
thin, warm, moist skin	dry, flaky, cool skin
frequent increase in appetite	lack of appetite
loss of weight	increase in weight
bulging eyeballs and unsteady gaze	tendency to expressionless gaze
occasional diarrhoea	tendency to be constipated
enhanced reflexes	hypaesthesia
disturbed sleep	sleepiness
slight trembling	stiffness in the extremities

One may thus say that the thyroid is the balancing and regulating organ between the inside (metabolism) and the outside (nerve and sense system), in the same way that speech may be said to be the balancing and regulating activity between within (feeling) and without (world). It is apparent that the thyroid has a particular relationship to speech, beyond its physical proximity to the larynx. It works particularly into the soul and spirit element in speech and what is audible in the flow of the voice in speaking. The thyroid reacts very sensitively to the relationships of tension in the astral body. That is why illness is often accompanied by vocal disorders or impairment of the speech instrument. The tongue and vocal chords are particularly affected by this.

The thyroid exercise regulates and harmonizes the functions of this organ in a very differentiated and effective way. In hardly any other exercise does Rudolf Steiner avail himself so comprehensively of the artistic principles of speech, and apply them for their therapeutic efficacy.

Structure of the exercise

At first sight, one is struck by the unusual length of the lines and of the whole text. The seven lines, of which each has a clear sentence structure in itself, should be practised several times a day, according to Rudolf Steiner's instructions. The elements of perseverance and commitment are clearly called upon here. In addition, the repetition of apparently meaningless combinations of sentences brings something calming toward the pole of the nerves and senses. The whole human being begins to free itself in the flow of speech and become more musical. The long drawn-out vowels, particularly in the first part of the exercise, support this releasing, flowing process, as does the frequent use of the richly vibrant consonant N. This sound in particular does the thyroid good, according to another remark of Rudolf Steiner's in the Workmen's Lectures.

> With the thyroid, it is true, one has to intervene occasionally, because it is extraordinarily hard to make the thyroid better through what I would call spiritual means; but even so it is possible to achieve positive results. They have already been achieved. If one has someone repeat things every day in a particular way, again and again, in a song-like way of speaking, then the thyroid actually recedes.[2]

In the last three lines of the exercise the language becomes condensed through the accumulation of consonants, while the tone spectrum reduces to the vowel E.

The sounds

In the first line the repetitions of the vowels A A – E E E E – I I I I stand out. Rudolf Steiner uses the vowel sequence A E I to introduce other speech exercises also (for instance the exercise Aber ich will nicht dir Aale geben). This sequence of sounds stimulates the will for speech, in that the soul is led forward from the back of the speech instrument, making its way from breadth into the directional. They are the principal vowels of the thyroid exercise. All three lie in the back part of the speech instrument and are in interplay between the metabolism (A: palate) and the nerve and sense pole (E/I: teeth).

The vowels E and I, which clearly predominate in this exercise and which also appear as the final vowels in most of the lines, are the two nerve vowels. The speaker thus alternates between the E which has a consolidating effect inwards on the flow of the nerves and the nerve process directed outward in the I. This encourages a delicate sensing between the unconscious and the conscious nervous system and creates balance.

The bright blood vowel A brings expansion and release for the one practising it. Then the nerve pole is taken hold of, moved through between calm and direction, and finally consolidated in the repeated E sounds. The first few lines, spoken in rather a calm, measured fashion, with their full, emphatic vowels, have a particular effect on the out-breath. The condensed consonantal quality brings agility and a quicker flow of the speech into the last few lines. Here it is particularly important according to Rudolf Steiner, to keep apart the final sound of one word and the initial sound of the next word when they are the same sound. The forces of the blood are stimulated thereby and the I practises gripping and letting go.

The measured, almost song-like vowels at the beginning of the exercise are complemented by the nasal sound N, with its wealth of vibration, which is able to free the voice from resonating in the head. The consonants then alternate chiefly between warm blown sounds (S, W) with their affinity to warmth, and distinctly contoured impact sounds (G, D, T, B), that is between the polar elements of fire and earth, spirit and matter. It is important to bring about a balance between these two and introduce mediating processes.

The speaker is called on here to be very agile in moving between the zones of the sounds. A strong element of will is brought into one's speech not only by the way the initial sounds in some lines alliterate, such as the W in the second and sixth lines; but also because the same sound sometimes begins more than one syllable in the same word. The almost dramatic alternation in the second line between W and G is calmed in the next two lines through the highly contoured impact sounds: heat is cooled down by form. Here the B in particular gives a protective mantle and the possibility to release by means of voice and breathing what has become blocked.

Again and again the consonants return to the teeth and tongue sounds. These correspond to the astral body which, in the last line in particular, is aired through, formed and brought into oscillation through R D T N, thereby reinforcing the calm pole of E through placement exclusively on the teeth. The consonants relate particularly to the pole of the nerves and senses and bring balance to the astral forces. This exercise teaches the speaker to perceive how they live within the different possibilities of their soul life and how to consolidate this by self regulation. In practising this exercise one imitates momentarily the task of the thyroid and gives it an example, as it were.

Rhythm

Although the lines do not follow a fixed rhythm, the longs and shorts are meaningfully integrated into the totality of the exercise. In particular, the change from falling to rising and from rising to falling rhythms creates caesuras for the consciousness and demands a similar agility to that needed in the transitions between sounds and the grasping and releasing of the different zones of speech. The unique character of the syllable repetition with which this exercise begins, underpins the measured, musical cadence of the first line. These are sound repetitions, through which the speaker is led on into the exercise in spondaic syllable stepping: An-an-/ ge-ge-/ benes ... The second line is entirely in a falling trochee. Although over the course of the exercise the beginnings of the lines tend to be short, this aspect has more the character of a prelude. The voice repeatedly finds and releases itself in a swinging, falling long syllable, or steps with the syllables.

The fact that repetition of the same vowels, consonants, beginnings of words, syllables and rhythmical elements is one of the principal structural elements of this exercise reveals its deep affinity to rhythmical life processes, in which the activity of the glands has its origin.

Dynamic

The exercise is based on its own dynamic, consistently supported by the artistic means mentioned above. Beginning in completely calm, vocalic out-breathing, the speaker is led into a rhythmic encounter with the sounds.

The first line leads us into the exercise like a majestic invitation in content and form. Experience shows that this line should be spoken in one single out-breath. One should take care that the unvoiced S at the end of Angegebenes goes over into the voiced S with which sieh begins.

The second line expresses itself in the courage and boldness needed to bring W and G together into a declamatory relationship. Wogenwind is directed strongly to the periphery. New strength can be gained by means of an intermediate breath after the word wenig.

From the periphery, the enfolding form of the B responds and leads back to the centre again, to T, to Tat: from prayerful devotion in the B to the concrete Tat. This line gives us a direct experience of the thyroid's task, which is to live in strong polarities. This line too should be spoken in a single breath; the little word und, being a conjunction, should be moved caressingly.

Then the opposite gesture comes again, handing over everything from G to B. In this fourth line the goal is always the last little word ab, in which the A is breathed completely into the cosmic enveloping gesture of the B. Here too it is particularly important to bear in mind the recurring consonants. Gib biegend die Gabe ab. The breath proceeds downward in great arcs.

In the dynamic of the exercise there must now be a consolidation and contraction. In a sort of positive defiance, the fifth line is spoken in a concrete and definite manner as far as kleben. At this point, the musicality of the exercise changes almost entirely to a sober consonantal quality. The repeated consonants need to be taken hold of strongly. Nevertheless, the voice must go through this contraction without fail and experience it, when it comes to Kasten kleben, possibly as something unpleasant. Whether one needs to take another breath before auch is, in our experience, up to the individual.

There now follows a liberation from this constriction in the sixth line: the speaker moves from the warm heaviness of the first three deeply intoned Ws, then sounding the Ws increasingly musically in a kind of outward spiralling right into the periphery as far as 'wird winzig,' in order finally to feel the consolidating power of the E streaming into them from the periphery. The damming up in this line, after which a new breath may be taken, intensifies once more the musical swinging into the periphery. Another breath may also be taken before the two brightly radiating words wird and winzig.

If this succeeds, the speaker experiences support from the placement of all the consonants at the teeth in the last line, and at the same time feels a calming consolidation in the repeated sounding of the E. From within, a declamatory appeal for deliverance; from without, streaming into us, a consolidation of the nerve stream.

The more we practise this intense drama consciously, the greater its effectiveness.

According to Rudolf Steiner, the slight pain in the area of the thyroid and larynx which can be experienced after speaking the exercise — one could also call it a heightened awareness — should be guided into the limbs and the skin. After the intense centring in the last line, it is surprisingly easy for the patient to free themselves downward and outward from the larynx, and feel a stream of warmth toward the periphery, which they then divert into the limbs and skin.

Gesture and content

Most of Rudolf Steiner's speech exercises are relatively meaningless as far as the content is concerned. The functioning of the artistic elements of speech, undisturbed by conceptual thought, can thereby be assured. In spite of the apparent meaninglessness of the short practice sentences, their imagery can help in implementing the steps of the exercises.

For this exercise, Rudolf Steiner gave indications, quoted earlier, for conduct to promote health in the soul, which fit the images in the exercise:

> Apart from this one should observe one's disposition, for instance whether one soon leaves off doing something which one has undertaken to do and which needs to be carried out regularly over a longish period; however it should not be something which one

does in response to external authority, but rather something one has decided on oneself. It is very good to keep at it and not leave off.

Then one should wean oneself of a certain indifference which one might experience toward some things which could actually concern one.

What is meant is not, for instance, considering something is beneath one, but rather complacency, lack of interest, perhaps even apathy.

The many elements of repetition have already been mentioned, including repeated practice of the text, which supports the patient's perseverance. Their attention is directed to what is prescribed and what is necessary. They gain courage for action and are called on not to let themselves be distracted by agitation, but to centre themselves before acting. Then comes the great arc of letting go, giving it away, emptying themselves entirely, so that kein Nickel (no nickel) is kept back. The blockage is released and is diminished.

These sentences, images and gestures lead the human being away from restlessness, self-reflection and any inclination to hold back and toward meaningful and considered action that is directed toward the world. Each of the first five lines consists of an imperative. In the last line the exercise culminates in an appeal to rescue (errette) through speech (redend) the saviour (Retter) of earthly speech (Erdenrede) and to resolve and stabilize one's pathological conditions. That means letting the thyroid become a functionally healthy neighbour of the larynx again, and integrating the astrally imbued process of speech into the sphere of life.

Summary

In a vivid way, Rudolf Steiner manages in this exercise to work therapeutically, through the medicine of speech, on all four parts of the human being. Through the length of the lines and frequent repetition of the text, the I is activated and one's perseverance enhanced. The voice is strongly challenged from the most diverse aspects to enliven itself and work healingly into the life processes, through taking hold, releasing, expanding, directing and supporting. The life processes are rhythmically enlivened through the numerous and differentiated repetition elements. The predominant nerve vowels I and E and the many dental consonants reveal that this exercise is particularly concerned with centring and consolidating the astral forces. Regulated anew, these are now integrated once more between the I and ether body. At the same time, the breath pole (slow speaking of vowels) and the blood pole (rapid speaking of consonants) are also addressed.

Experience shows that this exercise works therapeutically in all cases where thyroid processes are disturbed; and also with some illnesses of the nervous system. The path taken by the speaker balances and harmonizes. Continually changing between different speech elements brings calming influences into the patient's movement and mobility into their calmness. There is significant therapeutic efficacy for both overactive and underactive thyroid conditions.

The exercise does, however, require careful introduction and accompaniment by the therapeutic speech practitioner, so that the many finely differentiated aspects can be worked on.

A Second Therapeutic Exercise: Richtig recht rechnen

DIETRICH VON BONIN AND RALF UNTERBUSCH

This exercise is taken from the case studies of the Clinical Therapeutical Institute in Stuttgart, which was founded in 1921. For three years, Rudolf Steiner gave advice for the treatment of patients there. The notes of the case studies, compiled by Dr A.G. Degenaar, contain the following entry.[1]

> Patient No. 111. Male, aged 21   July 13, 1923
> Has been suffering for two months from apical catarrh and a heart condition. He is very run down, mainly through malnutrition.
> Dr Steiner: 'Above all else, you must rest for two hours daily, in addition to your usual night-time sleep, so that you do not overexert yourself. On no account do any physical work; that is out of the question. In addition you must do proper speech exercises, in which you always try to breathe as deeply as you possibly can.
> Richtig recht rechnen richtet ruhige Rippen rastlos zurecht.
> Leben liebt Lehre, Lehre liebt Leben.
> Mut machen mir mutige Menschenmassen.
> Do the three exercises one after the other, to adjust the astral body, which has become far too weak recently. — Externally arsenic.

No further indications are available. Christiane Starke, a teacher of speech formation In Bingenheim in Germany, knew this patient, who was then 21. He described to her how the first part of the exercise took hold of the lung, the second part more the digestion, and the third the forces of courage. The meaning played a part, he said.[2]

Before the advent of X-rays, the concept of apical catarrh was regarded as a typical initial symptom of pulmonary tuberculosis. It involved an apical lung process of inflammation and catarrh (for instance bronchitis, infiltrate with collateral oedema, and so on).[3] It is interesting that Rudolf Steiner did not initially aim to treat the ether body of this patient, who was undernourished, strongly affected by the initial stages of pulmonary tuberculosis and suffered from a heart condition; nor did he suggest that the ether body was weak. He said that it was the astral body that was weakened and that the latter should be reinvigorated by alternating rest (at least two hours daily) with speech exercises.

In such a diagnosis, further light is shed on the aetiological problem in the makeup of the human sheaths by a comparison with the eighth case in Steiner and Wegman's book Extending Practical Medicine. There the case of a 34-year-old female patient with goitre, apical catarrh, gastritis and anaemia is presented, demonstrating a remarkable conformity with that of the patient mentioned above.

> The patient reveals a highly atonic condition of the astral body. The I-organization is thus held back, as it were, from the physical and ether bodies. The whole life of consciousness is permeated by a subtle, dull drowsiness. The physical body is exposed to the processes arising from the ingested substances.[4]

This last characterization corresponds to one in the first Medical Course, Introducing Anthroposophical Medicine, concerning an imbalance in the ether body, which is called 'hysteria' there, and referred to as the basic constitution underlying pulmonary tuberculosis. In therapeutic speech, declamatory texts have been found worthwhile.[5]

The case presentation continues:

> These substances are thereby transformed into parts of the human organization. The ether body in its coherent vitality is too strongly muted by the I and the astral body; ... All the bodily functions thus have to take a course whereby they come into disharmony with one another. Inevitably the feeling arises in the patient that she cannot hold the functions of her body together with her own I. This appears to her as a powerlessness of the soul. Hence she says she is more psychologically than physically ill. If the powerlessness of the I and astral body increases, disease conditions must arise in various parts of the body, as is also indicated by the different diagnoses. Powerlessness of the I expresses itself in irregularities of glands, such as the thyroid* and the suprarenal; also in disorders of the stomach and

intestinal system. ... Most characteristic is the following: owing to the powerlessness of the I and the astral body the need for sleep is partly satisfied during waking life, the patient's sleep is therefore lighter than a normal person's. ... In the inner organs the powerlessness of the I first expresses itself in the lungs. Infection of the apex of the lung is in reality always a manifestation of a weak I organization.

If we examine the medicines prescribed for the patient in Arlesheim and the patient in Stuttgart, they are autumn crocus (Colchicum autumnale) and arsenic. Rudolf Steiner speaks in several places about arsenic and its effects. It has an energizing effect on the astral body in general and bolsters its influence on the physical body; it also harmonizes the astral body's relationship to the ether body and physical body.

Autumn crocus is a cardinal remedy for goitre. We are concerned here with an 'atonic condition' of the astral body which has to be worked on, and to which the remedy corresponds: 'We have discovered that Colchicum autumnale has a powerfully stimulating action on the astral body, notably on the part that corresponds to the organization of the neck and head.'[6]

In both cases it was a matter of 'adjusting', of strengthening the astral body. For the situation in Stuttgart, Rudolf Steiner prescribed rest, a speech exercise and arsenic, applied externally. If Martha Hemsoth were then already working at the Clinic in Arlesheim, the Arlesheim patient would presumably also have been prescribed therapeutic speech.

The significant remark that apical catarrh was actually always an expression of a weak I organization gives us occasion to examine further the application of speech exercises for weakness in the I organization and astral body, particularly in the upper part of the organism.

In the Speech and Drama Course, Rudolf Steiner locates the speech impulse in the 'astral body modified by the I'.[7] When the human being speaks, the modified astral body takes hold of the sound-forming forces of the ether body and lets the impulse which has thus been formed resound in the physical body. The essential aspect is the nuance 'modified by the I'. From within the I, conscious speech formation takes hold

---

* Rudolf Steiner gave a specific speech exercise for goitre patients (An Angegebenes ...), which provides further evidence for speech formation being indicated in such cases. Comparison of these cases reveals the consistency between the situation in the human component parts of the patient in Arlesheim, the patient in Stuttgart and also in the different patients suffering from goitre for whom the exercise An Angegebenes was given.

of this impulse, gives it tone and life, and forms and moulds it right into the body.

It is thus not hard to understand why therapeutic speech is particularly indicated in cases of a weakened I and an 'unadjusted' astral body; particularly the exercise which we have been looking at: Richtig recht rechnen ...

Our late colleague Agatha Lorenz-Poschmann made a commendable study of this exercise. She placed it at the centre of a whole book on therapy through speech formation, so we will confine ourselves here to only a few aspects of the exercise. It begins with an in-breathing imbued with the I-organization, an opening-up to take in the quality of the R, in order then to guide R – Ch (blown sound) – T (impact sound), light-imbued, from above downward, to the earth as it were, helped by the movement of the sounds. The R lives out of the founts of the in-breathing. The L lives in and with the living will-imbued flowing of the out-breathing. It gives the possibility to take up the forces of weight and of matter and transform them into flowing life.

This gesture is then elaborated more particularly, through the vowel sequence E – I – E (in the line Leben liebt Lehre ...), or strength — light — strength.

In the middle part of the exercise, there is an intensification through repetition of the words in the opposite order.

The nature of M lies in saying yes to the world with body and soul. It penetrates deeply into all with its warm, nasal intonation. Voice and breath unite themselves most intensively into a flowing unity.

The sound-movement M – U – T makes this coming-to-oneself very clear. When the penetrating power of the M is completely taken up in a deep, warm U and kept going as far as the impact sound T, then the human being has come to themselves and arrived in the world. Above and below (here, upper lip and lower lip), within and without, in-breathing and out-breathing are all striving for balance.

The fairy tale of the Star-Money conveys the path of this exercise in a beautiful metaphor. At the end of the tale, after all the hardships of a devoted life, the silvery bright stars fall from heaven to earth and give the Star-Money child a new dress. In the same way the R, with its star-like qualities of light and air, leads the way from the upper to the lower human being. Then the Star-Money child gathers the money into her newly received garment, just as the L of the exercise releases the voice from weight, transforms it into liquid gold and leads it into the river of life.

The Star-Money child thereby becomes wealthy for the rest of her life, just as in M the voice, filled with inner warmth and new soul courage, flows affirmatively into its own breath stream.

For decades this exercise has been applied in different ways in therapeutic speech, and has demonstrated its effectiveness in terms of what is presented above.

A Third Therapeutic Exercise:
Ich atme Kraft des Lebens

Dietrich von Bonin and
Barbara Denjean-von Stryk

The origin of this exercise has been generously conveyed to us by Willi Kux,[1] who was the original recipient. It is worded as follows:

> Ich atme Kraft des Lebens
> In Luft verhaucht der Hauch
>
> I breathe in power of life
> In air the breath breathes out

The speaker should use up all their breath in the first line, then hold their breath until they have repeated the line silently to themselves three times, before breathing in deeply and speaking the second line, again using up all of their breath. They should then immediately take another deep breath and repeat the whole sequence up to seven times. It has since been used by many practitioners of therapeutic speech formation and shown its outstanding efficacy. It is also connected to a few similar-sounding texts by Rudolf Steiner, particularly:

> Ich atme die Kraft des Lebens aus den blauen Fernen
> Ich veratme das eigene Selbst in die blauen Fernen
>
> I breathe the power of life out of the blue distances
> I breathe out my own self into the blue distances

and also:

(Breathe in and think) Die höchste Kraft der Natur strömt
mit dem Atem in mich ein.
(Hold your breath) Alle Kraft ruht in mir.
(While breathing out) Ich ströme aus alles Gute,
dessen ich fähig bin.²

(Breathe in and think) The highest power of nature flows,
with my breathing, into me.
(Hold your breath) All power is at rest in me.
(While breathing out) I stream forth all the good
I'm capable of.

In contrast to these texts, which are presumably concerned with pure breathing exercises guided by thought, Ich atme Kraft des Lebens is a speech exercise. When comparing them, it becomes clear how, through the rhythm of the iambic trimeter and the clear structures of sound and image, the conceptual element recedes and artistic speaking is promoted. In this way, the breath can take its start predominantly from experience and less from consciousness. This is important, especially for the in-breathing which, through overemphasis in the present time on the pole of the nerves and senses, has forfeited objectivity and thereby depth. This can only be remedied through a speech-oriented in-breathing, rather than one oriented toward thinking.

The exercise begins with the vowel I, the sound which raises the human being to the upright, gives them direction, strengthens the power of conviction and stimulates joy and strength in the speaker. Through the following Ch, this light is taken over by the out-breathing, and lives likewise in the concept of the word Ich, 'I' as in 'I am'. In order to be able to speak this with all one's heart, the breath goes deeper than usual. It can then expand in A along with the soul that is now upright and awake, let itself be energized through the consonants, and finally become consolidated in E. This first line begins with a mood similar to that of the major in music; this mood then guides the human being back into the body through the vowel sequence from A to E: the light which has been taken in is now incarnated. The consonants are very balanced; every element is represented. The out-breathing is stimulated particularly through the vowels, and facilitated through the blown sounds.

Remaining in a breathed-out state needs to be accompanied by the therapist in a particular way. On the one hand, air should not flow in unnoticed through the open lips or the nose; but neither should persisting in the breathed-out state lead to a condition of tension or cramping. On the contrary, breathing out means devotion here; the speaker should breathe away muscular tension, releasing it, and inwardly repeat the first line in calm relaxation. When breathing in again, it is absolutely essential to have the second line present in one's mind and to take hold of the exercise's second I (In Luft verhaucht ...) as one breathes in. It is not good if this deep in-breath after holding the breath has nothing to take hold of, nor if it is obstructed while the speaker considers what comes next. It is not air hunger that should characterize this exercise, but the pressing need to continue speaking.

This second part of the exercise also begins with the I, but then receives a darker, fuller colouring through the blood vowels U and Au. It appears lighter and more mobile, through both its content and the consonants used, and less imbued with will. Blown sounds and the R increase, and warm the sentence through in a particular way.

Comparing the two lines shows a path from light-filled breath to breath that is increasingly mobile and warmed-through. The path from light into warmth is that of incarnation. The speaker then repeats this seven times. Each time joy needs to be reawakened, so that the I breathes the forces of life. Joy itself is an important factor in healing when an illness has come about through irregular intervention by the I.[3]

Incarnation is supported in a particular and unusual way by remaining in the breathed-out state. With every in-breath, the I moves through the lungs into the blood; the astral body also unites itself more deeply with the body. In the out-breath, these two elements of the human being are released out of the body a little. If breathing in is prevented, a kind of vacuum arises, which results in the I and astral body being 'sucked' into the body with the following in-breath.

Willi Kux also spoke of an aid to incarnation. When the exercise is spoken, the declamatory character of the first statement is immediately apparent: Ich atme Kraft des Lebens (I breathe the force of life), going from the self, the I, to the world; as is the recitative, descriptive style of the second statement: In Luft verhaucht der Hauch (In air the breath breathes out). The first statement is repeated silently to oneself, impresses itself deeply. It brings forth the joy of anticipation for the renewed in-breathing — now experienced very consciously.

In therapeutic practice the exercise has proven particularly helpful for acute and latent forms of hyperventilation.

The contraindications need to be considered. These affect patients with high blood pressure, above all people of a pyknic build, for whom the exercise, if done at all, must be applied only with great care. The exercise has shown itself to be useful — albeit very challenging — with asthma, as well as for lightly-incarnated people, in cases of iron deficiency, and in states of weakness after being confined to bed.

This exercise, as were the ones presented above, was given after the esoteric school ended with the First World War, which makes it clear that, in individual therapeutic contexts, Rudolf Steiner gave exercises with an indication concerning the breath even after that time. The 1908 esoteric lesson, printed in connection with Willi Kux's essay, reveals the comprehensive context of such a measure. The following is said there in connection with breathing out followed by holding the breath:

> When humans inhale, then the forces of the I become active, the forces that connect them with the powers of the universe, the forces that radiate outward from the heart. And when humans exhale, and when they hold their breath, then those forces of the I become active, which push toward the middle point, toward the heart, and create for them there a solid centre.

If one works at the exercise systematically and accurately one will be able to experience this 'and create ... a solid center' in the region of the heart.

Because of its comprehensive context, we have printed the 1908 esoteric lesson in its entirety. In it Rudolf Steiner goes into past and future conditions of humanity; at the end of it he places breathing and its conscious regulation in this context. It also becomes clear from this presentation how much awareness of the responsibility involved is called for when dealing with such exercises.

Reminiscences of Rudolf Steiner

WILLI KUX

In mid-1924 Marie Steiner wanted to include in a eurythmy performance one of the highlights at that time, the Ariel scene from the first Act of Part 2 of Goethe's Faust. This scene with Faust's great monologue, 'The pulse of life is beating, fresh and lively,' was particularly impressive. Faust was played by the multi-talented Dutch musician, Jan Stuten, who was living in Dornach at the time. He had also written some brilliant incidental chamber music for it. He was powerfully built, and had a resonant, manly voice. Many knew him as a superlative Adam in the Oberufer Paradise Play, which was regularly performed during the Christmas season under the direction of Rudolf Steiner. Stuten was ill and unable to perform. Marie Steiner, however, still wanted to include this scene and immediately started looking for a replacement. She thought of me. I had been at the Goetheanum in Dornach since Christmas 1923, in order to study eurythmy alongside my brother Ralph. For the task proposed for me, playing Faust in this scene, I lacked maturity, a speech training and experience on the stage. I therefore became caught up in a whirl of training and performing activities. I was a scrawny young man just turned 22 who had escaped from famine-stricken Germany.

To understand this tragi-comical situation one needs to know that only a few arty types lived around the Goetheanum at that time. Everything had to be carried out as well as possible with whatever talent was available. To this extent there was a certain similarity to the time of the premieres of the Mystery Plays in Munich, which were performed mostly by amateurs. That was only possible because someone of the calibre of Rudolf Steiner helped with and inspired everything.

I had just managed to learn the text of the mighty monologue. Marie Steiner worked with me untiringly every day, to regulate my speech organism and make it flexible. Eventually, at Marie Steiner's request, Rudolf Steiner spoke the monologue for me. Immediately it became clear that this was Faust! In the core of my being I was gripped by the might of his speech and his dramatic power. All the might of the awakening Faust's hopes and desires, the deep disappointment of this man who was almost dazzled, and the superhuman grandeur of his renunciation, became living sound and eloquent gesture in the countenance and the arms and hands of this unique personality.

None of this was any help; I only became even more worried. It became ever clearer to me that I was not yet up to such a task. I felt like a small boy in his father's coat that was far too big. As the day of the performance came nearer and nearer I was filled with despair. I could see the respected founding Council of the General Anthroposophical Society sitting in the front row, with Rudolf Steiner at their head, his eyebrows raised. I was standing or lying on the stage (I did not need to act Goethe's stage direction: 'Faust lying on the flowery sward, tired, restless, trying to sleep': I was living it). I was visibly losing weight, as far as that was still possible, and had lost the last colour from my cheeks. Marie Steiner, who had noticed this, was sympathetic and concerned. She asked during a training session whether I was ill, if I needed anything. I told her that years before I had had so-called apical catarrh, as a slight attack of tuberculosis was called in those days. However it had cleared up. One day, as we were having another big rehearsal with the whole roundelay of elves, and with Ariel and the orchestra, it was getting on for midday. Marie Steiner was untiring and implacable as she directed the rehearsal in the big hall of the joinery. The podium, from which in the evenings Rudolf Steiner held the mighty karma lectures, had been dragged into the middle of the workshop and provided with two wicker chairs. Marie Steiner was enthroned there like a commander, dispensing her direction, often conceived in the moment from her utterly artistic nature. My forehead broke out in sweat; gradually my own voice began to sound like that of a stranger, resounding in the room as from afar.

Around lunchtime Rudolf Steiner used to come over to the joinery hall from his studio to meet Marie Steiner and go with her for lunch, which they took in a little room behind the stage. Rudolf Steiner's forces, which had been stretched to the limit while consolidating the ailing and enfeebled Anthroposophical Society, alongside his comprehensive spiritual research activities, needed considerable nurturing. For that reason they did not go down to Villa Hansi, where Rudolf Steiner lived.

It was lunchtime and Rudolf Steiner came into the hall. He never arbitrarily interrupted when work was in progress, but would sit down beside Marie Steiner and carefully observe what was unfolding before him. Marie Steiner often took advantage of these providential moments to ask for eurythmy forms for the music in future performances. George Metaxa, who was Greek, and frequently played for eurythmy, would sit down at the piano to play the music. Someone would bring Rudolf Steiner a large drawing pad, which he would lay on his knee and on which he would at once draw the eurythmy form, in one continuous movement, while the piano music was played. We eurythmists and the others present thronged round him with great interest to see better. With great delight we followed the birth of a choreography which expressed the innermost essence of the music, as his delicate yet strong hand incredibly effortlessly conjured it onto the paper. When he had finished, he would show the completed form to us, usually with a child-like, pure joy in creation; he also gave indications for the dress and veil colours, and the sequence of coloured stage lighting. Being allowed to experience the creativity of such a great, universal artist was an unforgettable experience.

Rudolf Steiner was now sitting beside Marie Steiner. She suddenly leant over toward him and explained that she was worried about the health of young Kux, who was on stage just now. Rudolf Steiner asked me to come down from the stage and approach him. Everyone fell silent and drew nearer, curious to see what would happen. I stood in front of him, while he looked at me calmly and lovingly with his warm, dark eyes which were unforgettably mysterious. If I remember aright, he laid his hand on my shoulder to reassure me. Then, after a moment of concentrated silence, he said, turning to Marie Steiner, 'Herr Kux is not ill, he is healthy.'

That was probably the shortest, best and most accurate check-up of my life! He looked at me again and continued, 'However, I wish to prescribe something for you. You can practise it, and it will certainly help you.'

Saying this, he reached into the deep pocket of his long, black coat and took out one of the small notebooks that later became so well-known — there are hundreds of them in the Archive of Rudolf Steiner's Estate. He often mentioned that what has been experienced spiritually can only be remembered when converted immediately into symbols or concepts and written down; this was also his practice. Doing this was enough to fix it in one's memory.

He now wrote something in the notebook, tore the page out and gave it to me, with the request that I read it aloud. Self-consciously, I complied. As his writing was remarkably clear and easy to read, I could read it immediately. I read the following two sentences:

> Ich atme Kraft des Lebens,
> In Luft verhaucht der Hauch.
>
> (I breathe in power of life
> In air the breath breathes out)

When I had read both sentences aloud, he said I should now read the first sentence once more while paying attention to the following: I must breathe in deeply, then use up all the air in my lungs while speaking the sentence. This I did. I then had to speak it again the same way, but at the end of the sentence remain completely breathed out, with empty lungs, for the time it would take to speak the sentence slowly three times in a row. When I had completed that to his satisfaction, I had to breathe in deeply again. (While waiting with no air in one's lungs, the urge to breathe in increases enormously. One feels like a diver under water, longing for the moment when one may surface and breathe in again.)

Then I had to speak the second sentence; as I did so, Rudolf Steiner made sure that I used up all my breath. At the end of the second sentence, I did not have to hold my breath, but was permitted immediately to breathe in again deeply in order to repeat the first sentence, in the way described above. When I had understood that, Rudolf Steiner said to me, 'Practise that every day, speaking the two sentences in the way I've shown you, seven or eight times in succession. That will help you.'

Once I has been practising it for quite a while, I realized that each sentence has three stressed syllables: the first with A and E; the second, U and Au. According to Rudolf Steiner's phonology, A and E promote the connection of the soul with the body; while U and Au promote a loosening or releasing.

Here I must add what in my opinion might have motivated Rudolf Steiner to give me this particular exercise.

After the burning of the first Goetheanum, all that was available to those keen to do eurythmy were the few practice rooms in the Joinery at the Goetheanum. During the day, of course, these were of course reserved for the performers, who were also teachers. (At that time there was still no eurythmy training at the Goetheanum.) So if a young beginner wanted to work their way into the mysteries of eurythmy, they had to practise either at night or at six o'clock in the morning. That is what my brother and I did. During this intensive practice in the mornings, I often became quite dizzy and had to sit down. My soul, which had barely returned from sleep, withdrew from my body once more, under the powerful effect of the eurythmic movements. It is known that Rudolf Steiner pointed out that the soul constitution of people receptive to anthroposophy is such that they do not enter with their soul so strongly into their body as others do who have a more materialistic view of life. Without doubt, Rudolf Steiner wanted to give me an effective remedy in this way. In his loving way, he was always prepared to help people most selflessly.

I was permitted to keep the piece of paper with the sentences written on it, to my great joy. I looked after it reverently and with gratitude, until it went up in flames during an air raid in the Ruhr during the war. It helped me become more consolidated in myself. It is a great help when there are difficulties with incarnating.

As far as the performance of the Faust scene in question is concerned, someone told Marie Steiner that a young anthroposophical actor was working at the city theatre in Zurich, and that he might perhaps be able to take on this role. He was approached and agreed to come. He played the part with the verve of youthful enthusiasm (as one might expect from a trained actor). He was Edwin Froböse; from that time he was united with Marie Steiner's life work. He remains active in Dornach to this day. [Froböse died in Arlesheim in 1997.]

Esoteric Lesson

Rudolf Steiner

Munich, January 16, 1908

Manuscript from Anna Weissmann

Our last esoteric lesson was concerned with the great lawful regularities of the spiritual life as they are revealed in the course of human evolution, with the great spiritual powers that guide what happens on the earthly plane and take over from one another in their guidance. Today we want to speak in a somewhat more intimate way about the laws of the spiritual life as they unfold within the human being.

Those who are engaged in an occult training are, in a certain sense, waiting, are seekers. They are waiting for the day when a new world will open to them, a world other than the one they usually perceive. They are waiting for the day when they can say, 'I see a new world: between all the things that I could perceive in space around me I see a profusion of spiritual beings that were hidden from me before.'

In order to become very clear about this you need once again to call up before your soul the seven conditions of consciousness that human beings in the course of evolution must pass through. The first state of consciousness that the human being had to pass through was a dull, dim degree of consciousness, in which the humans felt themselves to be one with the cosmos; this state or condition is called Saturn existence. In the Sun existence the compass of consciousness decreased, but it became all the brighter. When humans then lived through Moon existence, their consciousness was similar to what we experience as a last remnant in our dreams; it was a dim consciousness of picture. Here on the Earth we have bright day consciousness, which will remain when humans on Jupiter raise themselves to picture-consciousness again so that we will have a bright consciousness of pictures. Humans will then raise themselves to two additional, higher states, the inspired and the intuitive. Thus our bright day consciousness stands between the dim picture-consciousness of the Moon and the bright picture-consciousness of Jupiter. And what the esotericist awaits, which will one day be revealed to him or her, is Jupiter consciousness. It will one day come upon each of you, one person earlier, another person later, depending upon ability, upon the degree of inner maturity.

However, Jupiter consciousness is already present in its initial seed-form in every human being. This future consciousness is already indicated in a very delicate way, but humans don't know how to interpret it. The esoteric life consists to a large extent in pupils learning to interpret subtle processes in themselves and in their surroundings. The Old Moon consciousness has not yet entirely disappeared, either, but is still present in its last remainder. The two conditions in present-day humans, in which in one case the Old Moon consciousness is still present and in the other case the new Jupiter consciousness is already present, are the feeling of shame and the feeling of fear. In the feeling of shame, where the blood is forced toward the periphery of the body, a final remnant of Moon consciousness still lives. And in the feeling of fear, where the blood streams toward the heart in order to find there a firm centre, the Jupiter consciousness is announced. Thus normal day consciousness swings in two directions.

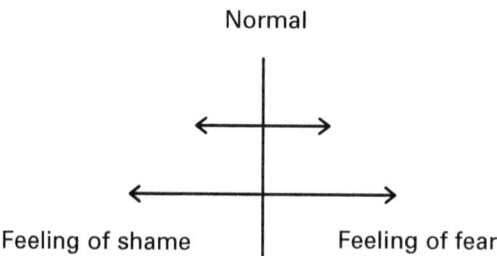

When we feel ashamed about something and our face turns red, we are experiencing something that recalls the Moon existence. Picture humans on old Moon. They could not yet say 'I' to themselves but rather lived in a dull, dim picture-consciousness entirely embedded in astral forces and beings, with which they felt themselves to be in harmony. Imagine, my sisters and brothers, if one day the feeling were suddenly to dawn on such a Moon-human: 'I am an "I." I am different from others, I am an independent being and all the other surrounding beings are looking at me.' From top to bottom the entire Moon-human would have been glowing with an incredible feeling of shame. Such a being would have sought to disappear, to be annihilated for shame, if it had been able to feel such a premature 'I-feeling.' Thus we, too, my sisters and brothers, when a feeling of shame overtakes us, would prefer to disappear, to shrink under the ground, to dissolve our 'I-ness.' Imagine how the old Moon-beings were embedded in harmony with the forces and beings in their surroundings. If they were approached by a hostile being they did not think about it but knew instinctively how to avoid it. They acted there with a feeling that, if they had been conscious, they could have expressed somewhat in the following way: I know that the order of the world is not arranged so that this wild animal will now tear me apart, but rather the harmony of the world is such that there must be means that will protect me from my enemy.

Thus old Moon-humans felt themselves to be in complete, unmediated harmony with the forces in the universe. And if an I-feeling had awakened in them it would have immediately destroyed this harmony. And as a matter of fact the I-feeling, when it began to permeate humans on Earth, did increasingly create disharmony with their environment. A clairaudient hears the universe sounding in a mighty harmony and when he or she compares it with the sounds that come from individual humans, then today there is with all humans a disharmony—with one person more, with another less, but there is a disharmony. And your task, in the course of your evolution, is increasingly to dissolve this disharmony into harmony. This disharmony arose through 'I-ness,' but it was instituted with wisdom by the spiritual powers who rule and guide the universe. Had humans always remained in harmony they would never have come to independence. Disharmony was instituted so that humans could once again achieve harmony in freedom out of their own power. This self aware feeling for being an I had to evolve at first at the expense of inner harmony. When the time then comes for Jupiter consciousness to light up and humans again arrive at a harmonious relationship with the forces of the cosmos, then they will preserve their self-aware 'I-feeling' into the new state of consciousness, so that humans will be an independent I and yet also in harmony with the universe.

We have seen that the new Jupiter consciousness is announced in the feeling of fear. However, it is always the case that when a future condition begins to appear before its time, then it is premature and not in the right place. This will become clear to you with an example. If one takes a flower, whose species should bloom in August, and brings it to blossom in a hothouse in May, then in August, when it actually should blossom, it will no longer be able to unfold a blossom; its forces will be exhausted and it will no longer fit into the conditions for which it was intended. And also in May it will have to fall into ruin as soon as it is taken out of the hothouse, because it does not belong in the conditions of nature of this time of year. It is exactly the same with the feeling of fear. It is not appropriate today and even far less in the future. What happens in the feeling of fear? The blood is pressed toward the centre of the human being, into the heart to form there a firm centre in order to make the person strong against the external world. The innermost power of the I brings this about. This power of the I, that works in the blood, must increasingly become more conscious and powerful. On Jupiter, humans will guide their blood very consciously toward the centre and be able to make themselves strong. However, what is unnatural and destructive about this today is the feeling of fear that is connected to this flow of blood. In the future that must no longer be allowed to be the case; only the power of the I, without fear, must be at work there.

In the course of human evolution the external world around us will become increasingly hostile. Increasingly you must learn to set your inner power against the world pressing in on you. But in so doing, fear must disappear. And especially for those who are undergoing an esoteric training it is necessary, unavoidably necessary, that they free themselves from all anxiety and feelings of fear. Fear has a certain justification only when it makes us aware that we should make ourselves strong; but all of the unnatural feelings of fear that torture people must disappear completely. What would happen if humans still had feelings of anxiety and fear, and Jupiter consciousness arrived? Then the external world would be set opposite the human being in a much more hostile and terrible way. A human being who does not cease to fear here will fall into one frightening horror after another there.

Already now this condition is being prepared in the external world. And this will be shown to humans even more clearly in that terrifying age that will descend under the regency of Oriphiel, concerning whom I spoke to you the last time. By then humans must have learned to stand solidly! Our present-day culture is itself creating the terrible monster that will threaten people on Jupiter. Just look at the gigantic machines that human technology constructs today with all its cunning! Humans are creating in those machines the demons that will rage against them in the future.

Everything that humans create today in terms of technical apparatus and machines will in the future come to life and will oppose humans in a terrible and hostile way. All that is created out of a purely utilitarian principle, out of individual or collective egotism, is the enemy of humanity in the future. Today we ask much too much about the utility of what we do. If we really want to foster evolution, then we must not ask about utility but rather we must much more inquire whether something is beautiful and noble. Everything that people do today in order to satisfy their artistic needs, out of pure love of beauty, this too will come to life in the future, but it will contribute to the higher development of the human being. But today it is terrible to see how many thousands of people are kept from knowing any other activity than those done for the sake of material utility; they are cut off from all that is beautiful and artistic all their lives. The most wonderful works of art should hang in the poorest elementary schools; that would bring boundless blessings to human evolution. Humans are themselves building their own future. We can get an idea of what it will be like on Jupiter if we clearly understand that today there is nothing absolutely good and nothing absolutely evil. Today good and evil are mixed in every human being. A good person must always say to him or her self that he or she has only a little bit more good than evil within, but is not at all wholly good. On Jupiter, however, good and evil will no longer be mixed, but rather humans will divide themselves into the entirely good and the entirely evil. And all that we cultivate today in terms of the good and the beautiful serves to strengthen the good on Jupiter, and all that happens only from the point of view of egotism and utility strengthens the evil.

So that humans in the future are a match for the evil powers, they must gain mastery of the most inner power of their I; they must be able consciously to regulate their blood so that it makes them strong in the face of evil but without any fear. The force that drives the blood inward they must have in hand. But also that other ability, to allow the blood to flow from the heart to the periphery, must not be lost to them. For the Jupiter condition will in a certain way also signify the return to Old Moon consciousness. Humans will again come into harmony with the great laws of the universe and feel themselves to be one with them. They will once again acquire the ability to flow together with the spiritual powers of the world, but not as they did on the Moon, unconsciously and dimly. Rather on Jupiter they will always retain their clear day consciousness and self-conscious feeling for self and yet live in harmony with the powers and the laws of the world. Disharmony will then be dissolved in harmony. And to be able to let themselves flow into the harmony of the universe they must consciously learn to let the inner power of their I radiate out from the heart. Thus they must be able to centralize the inner power of their blood when an enemy approaches them, and they must also be able to radiate them forth consciously. Only then will they be equal to future conditions.

Those then who strive for inner development must begin already today to get these forces gradually more and more under their control. They do this by learning consciously to inhale and exhale. When humans inhale, then the forces of the I become active, the forces that connect them with the powers of the universe, the forces that radiate outward from the heart. And when humans exhale, and when they hold their breath, then those forces of the I become active, which push toward the middle point, toward the heart, and create for them there a solid centre. Thus pupils are learning already today, when they consciously carry out their breathing exercises in this sense, gradually to become master of the forces of their I. However, no one should believe that he or she is allowed independently to undertake such exercises, if he or she has not yet received any instructions for them. Everyone will receive them at the proper time. However, even for those who are not yet doing any exercises, it is never too early to familiarize oneself with the meaning of these exercises and to acquire an understanding for them. Later these exercises will be all the more fruitful. Thus, my sisters and brothers, you should always get more understanding even for the subtle processes within yourselves and in the entire universe, and gradually grow into future periods of human evolution.

3

Aspects of Speech Formation

Upright Walking, Speech Movement, Eurythmy

GISBERT HUSEMANN

The whole and its parts

In the year 1887, Heinrich von Stein gave lectures in Berlin on the aesthetics of German classicists. (Rudolf Steiner's PhD, which he gained in 1891, was supervised by him in Rostock.) In one of von Stein's lectures on Goethe's approach to the natural sciences, he says, 'We differentiate a pear tree from an apple tree by its form, even from a distance from which we cannot distinguish blossoms, leaves or fruit. The pear tree is generally longer, the apple tree rounder; the shape of the former resembles a pear, that of the latter an apple.' Comparison of the whole with the parts reveals the same formative tendencies.

Von Stein made the further discovery that the leaves of both trees are also formed in a corresponding manner. The same 'form tendency' is maintained, with transformations, throughout the parts of the tree, 'from the root to the place where the twigs begin — and again where the leaves are formed. It is active ultimately in the circulation of the fluids through which the ripening fruit is formed.'[1] In this way, the 'unity of the formative forces' could be seen, even 'quite coincidentally' and even through merely 'superficial' observation. Von Stein advocated Goethe's ideas on metamorphosis in an age which was strongly averse to Goethe as a naturalist.

We will now attempt to apply this principle of seeing the whole in the part to an example from a study of the human being. We shall reflect the larynx, as a part, in the mirror of the whole form. The latter will therefore be described first.

The upright movement of the human being

When the human being gets up in the morning from a position of rest, various muscles come into play. After a brief holding of the breath which precedes every effort, the straight muscles of the abdomen tauten and contract, from the pubic symphysis, via the thorax, as far as the neck. This muscular pull would open the lower jaw, and the head would be lowered forwards; however, the jaw muscles simultaneously contract and lift the lower jaw; and the neck muscles leap into action and hold the balance from behind, so that the head is the first to be lifted. We do not notice any of this. Without knowing how it will turn out, we bite, in a manner of speaking, into the new day. The jaw muscles are only parts of a chain, which begins at the pelvis and continues via the sternum and the neck muscles. The movement is taken up by the neck muscles, through the mouth, via the gullet and the speech organs. In response, the pull forward is balanced from behind; the head, after all, should not hang down (like an animal's) but be held upright.

The hip joint

The back muscles are responsible for the further raising of the torso into the upright from a sitting position. We may easily distinguish a lower, a middle and an upper region. In the lower region is the gluteus maximus. From the head and neck of the femur it overlaps the hip joint; it attaches to the strong, semicircular iliac crest. Uprightness came about, far back in the mists of time, in both hip joints, when the joints were not yet fully formed; it still happens there today. The human being raises the body from sitting, around the lateral axis of the hip joints. The hip joint is the biggest joint with the greatest lifting capacity and resilience, and with the strongest muscle (gluteous maximus); the sciatic nerve, which is the thickest, goes past it into the legs. This is anything but coincidence, for in this joint the weight of the body is drawn up and lifted; to bring this about, the feet must be firmly on the ground. Children and people carrying heavy burdens demonstrate how the first thing that the feet do is seek the right stance for the burden. The weight of the body is shifted upward until the eyes can look straight ahead and upwards. The animals look down toward the earth; apart from the birds, only the human being can see the stars.

Further muscle chains

The musculature of the hip does not work in isolation. We now need to look at the totality of the muscles involved. The muscle fibres of the gluteus continue in the same direction on the opposite side; with this, we reach the middle region and the broad back muscle, the latissimus dorsi, which is the muscle with the greatest surface area.

As the figure shows, the muscular pull of both hip muscles is first taken up by a sinewy (muscle-free) plate. Once the muscle power has passed through the aponeurosis, it runs into another muscle, which takes up the direction and determines where the latissimus, and with it the whole chain, ends on both sides: at the upper arms. Coming from two sides, two great muscle chains cross over each other near the upper edge of the pelvis and push onward. Because the gluteus continues as far as the lower leg, they actually begin below the knee joint and end on the opposite side at the upper arm.

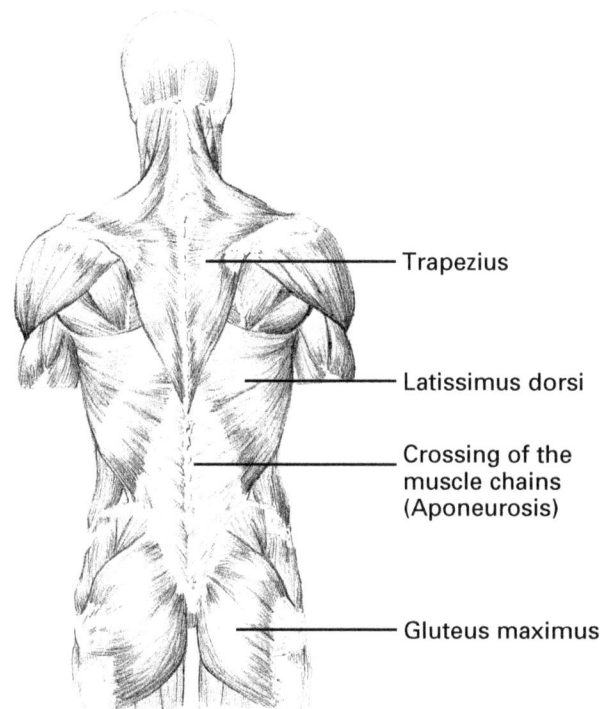

Back muscles (After D Welch)

The knee joint, the hip joint, the spinal column as the line of crossing, and the upper arm in the shoulder joint are integrated from behind on both sides into one of the muscles, whereby the individual muscles subordinate themselves to the pull of the whole.

We are thus enfolded from behind by two large, crossed bands of muscle, to which cling the numerous longer and shorter back muscles from deeper layers, and which set the body vertically on the earth through their joint activity.

Two details should be given particular attention. The precision of the blueprint, from the whole down to the parts, is revealed through the fact that the gluteus begins at the greater trochanter at exactly the height of the point of pivot of the hip joint. The muscle becomes, purely topographically, the circumference of the loaded centre of the joint, affecting it tangentially. In this respect, this joint becomes an image of the polarity between the centre of the earth and the cosmic periphery. The moved form becomes a part of something greater still. The polarity of the earth and the cosmos is embodied in the hip joint as an image of centre and periphery and has become the mechanics of the joint. The world of cosmic and earthly forces is reflected in the movement human being.

The other detail consists in the basic alignment of the body's centre of gravity just in front of the crossing point of the bands of muscle. Where they cross, the streams of muscle to do with uprightness run precisely behind the centre of gravity of the whole frame. The muscle chains raise us up and then continually monitor this posture we have attained in its fragile balance; for the centre of gravity lies above the points of support in the hip joint. In the animal, by contrast, it lies below the points of support (horse, penguin, duck). A fundamental difference between human being and animal becomes apparent through the conditions of balance. The animal, with its four legs, lives through its body in a stable state of balance with the earth, indeed the whole world, no differently to a chair or table. The human being stands out from all the animals through the fact that his balance comes about in and through the organism: the centre of gravity is lifted upward and outward in opposition to the forces of the earth. The human body exists physically in a fragile state of balance (which has moral consequences and consequences for the soul).

Rudolf Steiner said, 'Everything that comes to expression in human speech and human thinking is intimately connected to these relationships of balance.' This will become even clearer later on.

What we have already seen as a principle in partial manifestation in the hip joint, is fully realized here for the whole figure at the centre of gravity. The anti-gravitational forces at work here[3] flow into the muscular pull, grasp the skeleton peripherally and tangentially in a pincer movement, as from the cosmos onto the earth, and bring the human being into movement on the earth. A description of muscles becomes a tracing of the ether body, for it is the latter that brings the muscular system into being.

When, as children, we play on a swing we exercise the muscle chains. What do we do? Our hands first have to grip the ropes of the swing tight;

this gives us the fixed point — in addition to the attachment to the beam above — given us by our feet when we stand. We straight away bend our torso deeply forward, and the bands of muscle in our backs stretch and extend in readiness. The centre of gravity is now behind and, with one fell swoop — the hands on the ropes have to hold tight — the bands of muscle are contracted, pushing the pelvis forward. The body is grasped from behind and hurled forward: the legs are stretched straight in the knee joint. The swinging that is achieved is the complete equivalent of upright movement. Instead of the feet, the hands are fixed; instead of the upright orientation, the extension of the hip joint brings about the swinging pendulum of the body back and forth. The whole body swings freely, like the breath in the lungs. And that is just what delights the child. The playground swing allows the child to experience, enlarged externally, what occurs between its own muscle-body and skeleton, and between its ether body and physical body.

Musical instruments have the same significance later on (from seven to fourteen) for that constituent of the human being that has to do with the soul; in a heightened way they allow the working of the astral body to be experienced. Of course, this practice has greater educational significance than that with the swing, which may be a game, but a meaningful game — an exercise for holding tight, courage and verve.

In the upper region we have to do with the trapezius. It consists of two triangles, the broad bases of which similarly abut on each other in a sinewy plate at the midline, along the spinal cord. The descending fibres, coming from the head, have their counterpart in the ascending fibres. Between them, fibres run diagonally between the shoulder blades. In the centre rises the thorn of the seventh (and last) cervical vertebra. The trapezius is able to fix the shoulder blades (with the help of other, deeper lying muscles) at any point on the ribcage, depending on which portions of the fibres contract to bring about what is most convenient for arm and hand movements. The shoulder blades are moveable, like the mobile, lower part of a crane. The arms and hands are moved to the desired position where they are to handle and take hold of things.

The larynx and its movements

If we compare the larynx, as a part, with the whole, we must bear in mind that we shall only be dealing with a section of the outer muscles of the larynx. The inner parts of the speech organs are reflected in different human organs.

The laryngeal muscles are some of the smallest in the body. They have no mechanical function for bodily movement; on the contrary, they have been freed from that and given quite other tasks. The whole larynx is made of sinewy muscle and is suspended from the hyoid bone; it can therefore swing freely. The whole speech apparatus is more or less tautened by the sternum, the mastoid process (behind the ear) and the lower jaw, according to the tone produced; it vibrates like the string of an instrument. Although the speech instrument appears to be like a string and as if created out of air, there are also formative tendencies in the muscles at the back of it that are subject to gravity, as we found earlier when looking at the whole. In the same way that the fruit mirrors the tree in concentrated form, we can also recognize in the larynx, as fruit, the tree from which it emerged. The larynx remains soft; the structures of the thyroid, cricoid and arytenoid cartilages show that ossification as a formative tendency is excluded from the larynx. This only happens in old age; the larynx remains youthful, even embryonic, throughout life. Its predisposition is to be like a seed. In line with such a state, the muscles are compressed into a very small space; they are not unfurled and have not become earthly. The functions of joints and muscles have nothing to carry other than tone and word in the air! Along with the tendency to ossification, gravity has also been kept away from the larynx.

The larynx as a reflection of the human form
We first become aware, in this comparison, of the oblique arytenoid. Its system of crossed muscle fibres repeats on a small scale the large muscle chains of the whole figure. The differences are considerable, the discrepancies revealing. In the larynx, there are not the interposed sinewy leaves which were so important mechanically. Sinew is dying muscle, it is absent from the larynx. The elements to be enfolded in the part are the arytenoid cartilage and the epiglottis; only two elements in contrast to the large number in the whole: pelvis, leg, spinal column, ribs and arm. In the part everything is smaller, because squeezed together. The tissues remain soft muscle; more solid tissues disappear. Joints do not guide movements, as in the skeleton; here there are displaced joints, as in the arytenoid cartilage for instance.

In the whole, the centre of gravity lay in front of the crossing: in the reflection in the part, the oblique arytenoid muscles bridge the gap between the two arytenoid cartilages (not visible in the figure), from which the vocal cords proceed forwards. There is a mystery concealed here: corresponding to the centre of gravity in the whole, we have here to consider the stream of air which rises from the lungs through the windpipe, passing through the vocal cords. The rising stream of air carries speech outward on its wings. In contrast to the downward drag of gravity in the whole, here the freely-swinging flow of speech asserts itself on the

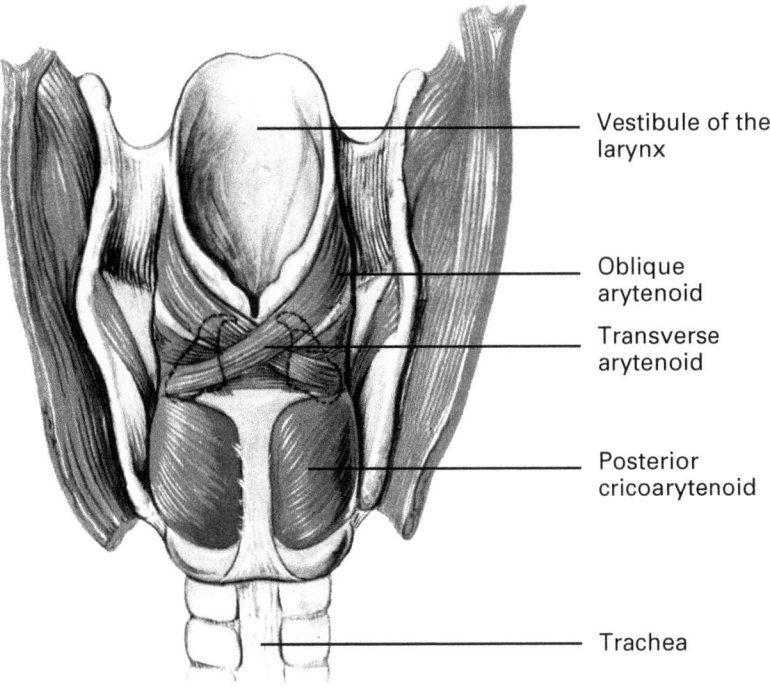

External muscles of the larynx, posterior view

out-breath, completely liberated from gravity; it wafts upward into the world. Seen in this way, centre of gravity and flow of speech are revealed as a polarity; this has already been described above in a different way.

In the larynx, the diagonal features of the trapezius appear directly below the fibres of the oblique arytenoid: the transverse part of the trapezius is reflected in the transverse part of the arytenoid. We saw how the trapezius can move the shoulder blades in sliding motions without a joint; the arytenoid cartilages are moved in a very similar way backwards and forwards in sliding movements with the cricoid cartilage as a base, even though connections in the form of joints are present. The speech parts of the arytenoid cartilages skim over the joints; they literally defy the connections to joints that would otherwise detain them. The organs are soft and the motion a kind of frisking flow, like waves moved by the wind of speech.

In the part, the three-sided shoulder blades are repeated and reflected by the arytenoid cartilages with their tetrahedral form. Attached to the shoulder blade in a ball-and-socket joint is the arm, ending in the hand;

similarly the vocal cords spring from the arytenoids. Further forward, however, they are fixed to the thyroid cartilage. The hand's dexterity and the finely graduated movements of the fingers are completely transformed into the acuity of modulation of the vocal cords' oscillations, monitored by the hearing. This modification is of the utmost significance: it shows that the movements of the malleable and muscular fingers are transposed into the element of music, that is inwards, through their being retained in the larynx. An internalization takes place in the soul's speech area, in that crucial physical movement potentials atrophy, whereby what is externally tangible disappears. As we go ever deeper, we come to a scaled-down movement human being, which at the same time has been lifted up into the soul element.

Lastly we shall consider the cricoarytenoid and the latissimus together. The muscle which runs from the cricoid cartilage to the arytenoid cartilage has the outer appearance of the gluteus. Just as the gluteus bridges the hip joint from the greater trochanter and becomes an erector, this laryngeal muscle runs to the muscular process of the arytenoid cartilage, drawing it back. What is the result? The vocal cords, which run forward, are opened by means of a typical lever action. In this respect, the erecting of the human figure has its musical and vocal counterpart in the opening of the glottis!

If we recall that the gluteus and latissimus chain begins at the upper arm, then upright movement (gluteus) and arm movements (latissimus) take effect in the movements of the glottis and in the oscillations of the vocal cords. If we hold our arms straight out in front of us and move them sideways, this movement in the whole is what the corresponding organs (arytenoid cartilage and muscles) do in the part when they open the glottis and the vocal cords oscillate, that is, when we speak. (The anchoring of the vocal cords is disregarded in this example, which illustrates their opening.)

We have seen that the gluteus acts around the diagonal axis of the hip joint; so too can the arytenoid cartilage be tilted and moved toward the cricoid cartilage around a diagonal axis. These minute tilting movements of the arytenoid cartilage, which come closest, even mechanically, to bringing about an upright posture, intervene in the tensioning of the vocal cords in a kind of fine tuning when greater precision is called for, as in singing.

In summary these comparisons and reflections of the whole in the part and vice versa are as follows: the larynx reveals posterior muscular features which evolve according to the blueprint of the whole form. In this respect, the speech instrument is a transformed movement human being in miniature. The whole is, as it were, the developed parent; the little larynx its fruit, like the child. The movement of speech develops, according to plan, from upright movement. Why does the limb human being remain silent and not go beyond mute gestures? Because its movements are too slow to be heard. The speech-movement human being has been speeded up many times over and the organs have been tensed up, so that they vibrate like musical strings and can thus be heard.

The movement of the larynx

Lastly I should like to draw attention to the phenomenon that directly shows the identity of the movements of muscles and speech in their basic approach: the breath is held for every muscular effort; and when we speak, we interrupt our breathing. We barely notice either. The result of heavy physical exertion is muscular movement; of the movement of speech it is audible words in the air. In the holding of the breath and in its interruption, both share an absolutely identical circumstance. One part of the pendulum's swing falls and gives itself over to gravity and muteness; the other part rises, and there is movement or resurrection as word in the air.

The prerequisite for both actions is a certain pulling oneself together inwardly, in body and soul. Physically, it is in the muscular effort. The narrowing of the glottis become a portal of soul space. Closed or drawn together, the glottis portal is burst asunder after holding the in-breath, by the increased pressure of the out-breath needed for each word. Once open, the path of speech is free. In the same way as with the breathing, an action dwindles and is dammed up, the vocal cords are fixed to the arytenoid cartilage, the narrowing of the speech is formed and mobility is intensified.

The vocal cords, like the fixed arms, have their hands in the remaining structures — the palate, teeth, tongue and lips — which, like the fingers on the strings of the lyre, engage with the stream of the air from outside and shape it. Conversely, the opening and closing of the glottis can, if anything, be compared to a wind instrument, a kind of 'wind-fiddle'. The aptitude of the voice and the speech instrument have some of the features of a stringed instrument, some of those of a wind instrument. Through the dwindling and reduction on one hand, and the enhanced mobility on the other, the whole malleable figure is transformed into oscillating airy forms or a resounding sculpture of air: the word of the human being.

An arm movement, energetically extending the arm and pointing, means, as mute gesture: here! The speech movement into which the gesture is transformed in the air, swings quicker and here! is heard. In the H we hear the aspiration of the breath, in the I the directed extension of the elbow right into the fingers, in the R the circling muscular swinging. In speech, the mute gestures of the plastic form of the whole human being are thus revealed, musically and in spoken form.

In the whole, we discussed the conditions of the centre of gravity and of balance at the place corresponding to the stream of speech in the part; for the centre of gravity is reflected in the larynx where we had found the rising stream of speech.

When we compared the muscles, certain modifications and metamorphoses became apparent. Now we must consider something new: the centre of gravity as opposed to the upward impetus of the air. They develop a radical polarity out of the physical body. The body bears the stamp of the self, the I, physically, insofar as the body determines the unstable balance. Equally, the I reveals itself in the flowing air of speech.

The state of balance, as the physical reflection of the I and as the expression in soul and spirit of the speaking I, lives within this polarity. This polarity has become a prerequisite for the I in the body. Relationships of balance form the foundation of the architecture of the body. Only with this fundamental requirement can our body become the instrument of the I. Insofar as the balance is unstable, that has to be put up with; insofar as it is determined by the body, it has been vanquished, and spiritually free self-determination has become the task of the human being.

The laryngeal and back muscles, which were found to be modifications of each other, are gradated between the polarity of the earthly centre of gravity and of the stream of speech. One pole is immersed in the darkness of the will, the other encounters the light of thinking. The movements of uprightness and of speech in between are a kind of colour spectrum of potentialities of movement.

Upright movement and speech movement, as instruments, become identical in the being of the I that makes use of the instruments; whether walking upright or speaking. Rudolf Steiner's remark applies here: 'In speech is the resurrection of the human being who has disappeared in gesture.'[4]

Visible speech: eurythmy

If we are clear about the movements of the speech human being, including those much more important movements which cannot be described outwardly as they are supersensible, then we can apply those tiny movements of speech back onto the larger movements. As movement they become mute, but in return they become visible. Visible speech arises, and hence eurythmy. Insofar as the task of art is to reveal higher, invisible laws, eurythmy is the truly human art; for it makes the inner human being that culminates in speech and the meaningful word, manifest and visible.

The significance of this art for higher striving in face of the decline in culture becomes clear from a quotation. If someone wants to penetrate the essence of a seed, they should say to themselves, while examining closely the circumstances and the role of the seed in the development of the plant, among other things: 'What is invisible (in the seed) will become visible.' The human being itself also has a higher, invisible nature with its roots in the spiritual. From the germinal nature of the larynx, words become visible through the art of eurythmy. In this respect, eurythmy becomes a visual schooling for the invisible; for, as a bearer of the word, it makes visible the higher nature of the latter from the sphere of the word. Peoples have drifted apart as language has separated them. In the visible word, they can find their higher connection again in the sphere of the word. As eurythmy goes through the human world of separated peoples, it receives the task to make visible for the individual spectator the universal power of the word. The silent yet visible alphabet from alpha to omega testifies to the unifying logos, which the bodies of the peoples have rent asunder in order to attain their I. The archetypal source of all languages appears on stage in eurythmy. Individuals are thereby enveloped in the artistic element of the visible word, transcending their national identity; they become oriented toward their higher being with its roots in the spirit. The significance for the future of humanity of the transformation of upright movement into the movement of speech lies in the latter's transformation into the visible speech of eurythmy. If the former was an ancient evolutionary process, the latter must spring from free, creative, artistic, social activity.

All human beings walk upright, but they speak in different languages. If the upright body itself becomes the revealer of the word, then languages are significant only as modifications of the primal language, which is revealed as silent, visible primal language. Eurythmy brings a new annunciation of the word to all peoples. Does this not mean that a new Christ-word is given us with this art?

Science, art and religion

Thomas Aquinas wrote a commentary on the Prologue of the Gospel of John. The final section bears the heading, 'In the Beginning was the Word.' In it Thomas gathers together all the concepts he has already utilized and briefly elucidates once more the concepts or images of Father, Son, Likeness, Word, Begetting and Radiance. They are intended to help in comprehending Christ. Thomas writes:

> It is necessary to advance from a great variety of sensory images
> to come to a cognition of the divine; one alone is not enough ... So

we call the Son by different names in order to express the fullness of His being, which cannot be apprehended in one alone. The name 'Son' indicates that he is of the same essence as the Father; the name 'Likeness' that He is not unlike Him in anything; the name 'Radiance' that He is equally eternal; and the 'Word' indicates the immateriality of the begetting.

Concepts such as Son, Likeness, Word are sensory images for the cognition of revealed, supersensible, religious facts. Thomas wanted to penetrate into the being of the Christ-Logos and understand it; he did not just want to believe and abandon cognition. In the two centuries after Thomas human beings turned more and more strongly toward knowledge of nature. A person like Raymond of Sabunde expressed the notion that one needed to read, not just in Scriptura Sacra, the Holy Scripture, (which was written by human beings), but he said one must also read in the Scriptura Naturalis, the Book of Nature (which was written by God). He suggested one should consider that what is written by human beings could contain errors, whereas a book written by God could not. He used Aristotelian and Thomistic methods and concepts in order to read in the Book of Nature.

We should now consider the question whether concepts and images, such as those mentioned by Thomas, can be applied to nature. The whole form of the body, with its forces of uprightness, suggests a relationship with the earthly force field. The body of the earth and that of the human being are related to each other. What they have in common is substances and weight. As a reflection of this form we have become aware of a scaled-down, germinal speech human being. We have seen a metamorphosis of the human being of limbs, a transformation with gains and losses. There is a polarity: weight and slowing down on one hand; weightless speeding up on the other. Outer atrophy cleared the way for the movement human being to carry out its movements with increased rapidity. Movements of weight shoot with scaled-down movements weightlessly into number. They resound. Intervals and musical numerical relationships arise and become mediators of speech.

One can find the part in its relation to the whole only if one has a rule with which the proportions can be measured. The yardstick of our comparative methods, with the modifications and metamorphoses that have been found and the polarity that is operative, is the archetype itself, the spirit, which eventually appears as the word; for the spirit marries the word with the thought, in the air.

The concepts used have been handed down from antiquity. In the Wisdom of Solomon (11:20) we read: 'But thou hast arranged all things by measure and number and weight.' Solomon speaks further of the 'might of his arm', with which God formed the world. Rudolf Steiner has revealed the measure of the world to be the original warmth of old Saturn; number is a reference to the pulsation of old Sun; creation took on weight in the stage of Moon, which has become further densified into our earthly matter in the Earth stage. When we recognize bodily reflections in this cosmic mirror, they attain a cosmic language. We realize that the upright walking and speaking human being has become an embodied image of the creative Trinity: the spirit creates with measure; the principle of the Son is active in number; while in weight the Father principle holds sway.

The movement of speech in the sounding of numbers is formed out of upright movement in the weight of earth; as the I lives in both, the word resounds as the measure by which it comprehends itself. The mirror in which these proportions appear is the same in which we found the archetype, between upright movement in weight and speech movement through number. The images which appear have expanded and spiritualized themselves right into the principles of world creation. We can draw them together once more into the part and condense them.

If one can think of condensed upright movement as something pliable and external compared with speech movement; and if one can hear the great sculpture inwardly speeded up into music, then one will also understand that upright movement and speech movement become one in the I. Did not Thomas say that the concept of the likeness applies between Father and Son? In the spiritual blueprint for creation, number and weight and oscillations and substances originally had the same frequency or ratios: the one was the likeness of the other. Substances were caught up in music. In that respect, like Father and Son, they were 'not unlike [each other] in anything.' In the blueprint for earth, they became separated. Our example was that upright movement united itself with weight, while speech movement leapt into number. Thereby they became separated. Both, although different, become one again in the speaking I. We can find this way of thinking in Goethe, 'What is paramount is the recognition of different things as identical.' In our example, the paramount is in the I. Religious concepts are thus related to the facts of nature like an archetype to its representations.

Comparison of the inner space of the larynx or 'etheric uterus', as Rudolf Steiner called it, to the physical uterus helps in understanding Thomas's notion of immaterial begetting. Comparing the I's attitude to the sense organs with its attitude to the speech instrument helps in understanding Thomas's Radiance. These are further tasks.

These comparative concepts and images are intended to show how the tools of cognition themselves change. If, as was the case with Thomas, reason penetrates into the Christ principle, it is liberated from the dogma which holds down our thinking. The I also feels liberated from scientific dogma. This dogma does not hold down our thinking, but rather keeps it on predetermined tracks to be accepted. What was self-evident to Professor Capesius, but incomprehensible to Dr Strader (in The Portal of Initiation, Scene 9), actually comes about: concepts change according to their eras. Just because of that, their contents are cognized ever anew and differently, and become effective for the cognition of existence and eternity.

Thomas sought to understand divine revelation; Goethe was driven by his urge for knowledge to seek in nature for the Son principle. He began by taking his bearings for reading in the book of nature, from the logos. He thus found the archetype as the central idea in organic chemistry. Rudolf Steiner's observed the following: In Goethe's worldview 'lies the beginning of what must come about out of Thomism with really only a change of front in the direction of natural science.'[5]

Our comparisons of concepts tried to show this metamorphosis, this change of front, with a few, fundamental examples. We saw how great seekers after knowledge shook hands with each other. Today, observations at the summit of clairvoyance can be seen in harmony with the valley floor of natural science on the basis of the methodology founded by Goethe and Rudolf Steiner. Herein lies the future task of Goetheanism.

> Very much can be won from Goetheanism. Eurythmy has been won, which makes use of the human being itself as a new artistic element and which seeks to open up a quite new source of art.[6]

This new source of art arose at the same time out of the new scientific trend. While the evangelist wrote, 'the Word became flesh,' in a complementary image, eurythmy expresses it thus: 'The flesh as an instrument of art becomes word.' The question we posed earlier, as to what kind of annunciation of the word we had to do with, can be answered thus: eurythmy is a new Christ Word, a new epoch of the logos in art.

A hallmark of the new scientific current is the multiplicity of relations which are subjected to this comparative reflection. What is joined together as a whole from its parts is apprehended by a discerning imagination which compares, eliminates, gradates and so on. In this discerning observation between whole and part, and of the parts in relation to each other, the artistic element in cognition comes into its own; for the element of proportion is inherent to any art, whether architecture, painting, music or poetry. None can dispense in their way with measure, that is the proportion of the part to the whole.

Like any other scientist, the Goetheanist proceeds from observable findings; they then seek to understand the part in the mirror of the whole and both out of their relation and proportion. The things themselves begin to clarify each other. Religious concepts can be applied with a new vitality.

Images, insofar as they merge into the archetype, are rooted in the world of the Father; every metamorphosis and polarity evokes the power of resurrection; and when the type comprehends what is individual and separate, the Holy Spirit is speaking. The aim of spiritual science becomes apparent: to reunite science, art and religion.

The Fourfold and Fivefold Nature of the Human Being

Dietrich von Bonin

Anthroposophy is a method of cognition, the concepts of which are applicable not only to the physical world, but also to the world which lies behind material manifestations. Our task is to verify and describe this applicability. My methodology will therefore be to try to take statements by Rudolf Steiner about our specialist area — therapeutic speech — as hypotheses, and to see how far these can be verified with our means of cognition. The phenomena of our field are everything that is contained in speech formation and in those of its applications that are accessible to me.

The basic hypothesis in our case is the structuring of the human being as follows:

We are confronted immediately by two difficulties which arise from

Spirit man	Intuition
Life spirit	Inspiration
Spirit self	Imagination
I	Waking consciousness
Astral body modified by I	Dreaming consciousness
Ether body modified by I, astral body	Sleeping consciousness
Physical body modified by I, astral body, ether body	Unconsciousness

this description: the three 'lowest' parts of the human being — physical body, ether body and astral body — never appear in their 'pure form'; only the I is really independent. Even the astral body is modified in the human being by the I; the ether body by the astral body and the I; while all the other parts of the human being manifest in the physical body indirectly and in different ways.

Otherwise the I is only aware of itself during its principal activities of perception and thinking. For normal consciousness, therefore, the phenomena in the lower members of the human being have to be understood by means of perceptible and comprehensible manifestations. The astral and ether bodies are susceptible of direct research only through supersensible consciousness. The physical body is perceived 'from without' and serves as a mirror for wide-awake consciousness. Its inner processes appear to be accessible to research, but are accessible only 'outwardly' in terms of what has been outlined above. Bearing in mind these basic limits to observation, let us now consider the phenomena of speech, in order better to understand the involvement of each constituent part of the human being in speech.

Our starting point will be the speech of the adult; we shall attempt to consider the development of the speech of the child from this point of view.

In that I speak comprehensible sentences, I am present with the activity of my I in thinking, in the content of speech. That I am able to make use of a system of a particular language is a capacity which is present in me. I have to acquire the content of a lecture; the language which is necessary to mediate this content to me, however, is to be found within me.

This leads us to consider further constituent parts of the human being, in which apparently this capacity to speak is present for adults. (Everything which is already present is not the active I itself.)

This appears to confirm a far-reaching remark of Rudolf Steiner's, which we shall pursue:

> Speech proceeds, not directly from the I of Man, but from the astral organism ... and it is from this astral body, modified by the I, that the impulse for speech proceeds ... For ... in ordinary everyday speech the single sounds are formed in entire unconsciousness.[1]

We must therefore seek this impulse for speech in the astral body — in its more conscious and less conscious regions. We shall first consider the development of speech in broad terms.

The first pre-speech utterances of the infant in the initial phase of babbling (up to about three months) are expressions of pleasure and pain, content and discontent. The impulse to expression takes hold of human beings in the purest and most primordial way when they scream. In the second phase of babbling up to the stage of the one-word sentence, sound-games predominate, in which all the sounds of the world's languages appear. As if by a miracle, consonants appear in the infant's soliloquy, which do not originate in the child's imitation of a language. Only around the age of one and after do children acquire words of their mother tongue and enter into spoken communication. At this point, the vowels are more clearly developed and the capacity of universal consonant formation becomes restricted to the sounds of the mother tongue. Children must pay for their increasing wakefulness through a certain limitation of the variety and universality of their stock of sounds, in favour of the elements and rules of their mother tongue. We can experience this struggle with speech through the children's utterances during their acquisition of speech; it continues throughout life.

The elements of the sounds are played with. The connection between sounds, syllables and conceptual content is still somewhat loose: 'back-mots, bot-mack, mat-bock, match-box.'

Thinking awakens gradually through language and speech; the following was said in bed in the morning (the child was used to having a mid-day nap).

'Get up, Hans; fetch mummy, fetch daddy ... mummy's still asleep ... daddy's still asleep ... is it mid-day? Is it not mid-day?' (24th month)

'I'm always saying so many things I don't understand. What does "disappoint" mean? What does "road accident" mean?'

'My shoe is pressing on my foot.' (The shoe is taken off.) 'It's not making an impress any more now.'

'We shall strike out on this path,' someone says. 'What, the path is going to be broken.'

'The cliff is crying.' (Waterfall)

What we take hold of during the phase of the one-word sentence is the mother tongue. We shall consider its significance later, when we look at the ether body; however we should bear in mind that it is called mother tongue. It is not called the I tongue.

We put on this language like a garment; as a gift which connects us to our people, but which also narrows us down. This language has to be taken hold of and shaped-through by the I.

Rudolf Steiner gave the original system of speech exercises to teachers of the Waldorf Schools, to help them make their speech their own anew and so become worthy to be a model in the realm of speech. The impulse to speech, which originates in the astral body, must be led by the I through all the layers of language, so that a language of the I may develop out of the mother tongue.

To summarize: before their birth, incarnating human beings are surrounded by the harmony of the spheres and by cosmic formative forces — the archetypes of the sounds. They experience them there as their inner world. Birth marks the beginning of a path through screaming, babbling, the one-word sentence and the mother tongue as stages of increasing focus towards the situation of beginning school, when by and large they will have mastered their mother tongue. From this time onward, without a new impulse, the mother tongue could increasingly restrict our soul-life for the rest of our lives, and represent something of a 'foreign body' in the life of the soul (in the sense of an untransformed, inherited element). The mother tongue would then have a hidden potential for causing illness and a laming of the I.

Through the acquisition of a foreign language, the portal to the language of humanity opens an initial chink. Herbert Hahn once compared this learning to the birth of a second soul within us. We become aware of the relationships of sounds; the ways of thinking of entire folk-spirits become apparent from how their concepts form themselves. An example is provided by native Americans on the west coast, who describe a spear as 'stick with a point for killing'.

The way of speech formation is the opposite. It is the way to the centre. Our own mother tongue is taken up anew on all levels and shaped consciously. From the level of the sentence and of the breath, via the syllable, to the power of sound-combinations and of the individual sound, their connection with our own body is researched and shaped. In this way, the I gains command over that previously unconscious part of the soul life, our mother tongue. A feeling of joy from consciously working with undiscovered possibilities fills us. Consciousness and the power to transform awaken in the face of resistance from the organization of the body and of language. Such experiences have a direct, health-bringing effect on all illnesses to do with our unresolved or inherited past.

We will now summarize the role of speech formation and that of foreign languages.

When people continue only with their mother tongue, they bear within them an untransformed part of their soul, which tends to fix and rigidify the life of soul.

Acquiring another language brings a new element into the astral body: a 'second soul', which broadens the horizon to take in more of humanity.

When speech is formed, the reworking of the 'foreign', inherited element itself begins. The archetype of language is discovered anew.

The process that has been described may perhaps be compared to the following. Childhood illnesses ensure that the inherited physical body and ether body are adapted to the incarnating individuality. For overcoming the limitations of the mother tongue we have speech formation, which places these inherited capacities at the service of the individuality, of the I. Both are warmth processes: fever in children's illnesses; enthusiasm in speech formation.

In order better to understand the role of the ether body in speech, we can take what Rudolf Steiner said in the course Eurythmy as Visible Speech as a working hypothesis:

> When the child comes into the world, the mother's milk is the best for the building up of the physical body ... And it is the mother tongue which, as we said yesterday, is the ether body, it is the mother tongue which develops and gives form to the ether body.

In what sense, then, is the mother tongue the ether body?

> Now if all the sounds of the alphabet were uttered from A to Z there would arise an etheric human being — only this etheric human being, born out of the human larynx and its neighbouring organs, would be imprinted into the air. ... Again the physical larynx is only the external sheath of that most wonderful organ present in the ether body, which is, as it were, the womb of the word. And we have before us that wonderful metamorphosis which I indicated while I was speaking about metamorphosis.
> ... The etheric larynx and its sheath, the physical larynx, are a metamorphosis of the maternal uterus. When speech is brought forth, what we have is the creation of a human being, an etheric creation of a human being.[2]

From these extracts it becomes clear that the level where the element of the sound in speech lives is that of the ether body. This realm of the sounds is revealed as a tremendously fundamental and robust structure, which all human beings have in common and which, as we have seen, is played with from the third month onward in the second phase of babbling without conscious intention, out of pure joy in the sounds. The issue of the metamorphosis of the uterus into the larynx is a research question, from the further elaboration of which we may expect significant therapeutic implications. Positive experiences have already been made in the treatment of dysfunctions of the sexual organs with therapeutic speech.

We shall now look at the involvement in speech of the different constituent parts of the human being, through the medium of the last sentence of a poem by Goethe, which we shall also come across later on.

> Seele des Menschen, wie gleichst du dem Wasser,
> Schicksal des Menschen, wie gleichst du dem Wind.
>
> Spirit of man, Thou art like unto water!
> Fortune of man, Thou art like unto wind!

Content	I, wide awake consciousness
Impulse	I in the astral body
Words	mother tongue, dream consciousness, astral body
Sounds	ether body
Sound production	physical body, placement of sounds, resonating chambers, etc.

An example:

S – E – E – L – E	feeling the tongue in the space of the mouth
S – E – E – L – E	gesture of the sound
Seele	gesture of the word (the ether body does not itself form words)
Seele des ...	gesture of the sentence
Line of a poem	contains more than just the content, a mystery

The mother tongue, tied to words lies in the region of the astral body: it must be transformed in speech therapy from out of the I.

The sounds are to be found within us in the region of the ether body; with the help of their archetypes we are able to improve and form our speech. The archetypes themselves are the forces of the planets and the zodiac. As an aid to practice, the eurythmy sounds can be formed and then felt silently. The sound is then spoken into this silent feeling; in this way it can draw ever closer to its archetype.[3]

The more beautifully speech arises as a sound-picture in the region of the physical body, the more the I is able to place the ether body's archetype of the sound in the service of the astral impulse toward speech.

Before we consider the fifth constituent part of our being, I shall draw together in a diagram what we have learned so far, placing it in connection with illnesses and therapy.

Constituent part	Element of speech	Speech disorder	Aspect of illness
Spirit self	Poetry	No access to poetry	Destiny aspect of the illness
I	Content of speech, the sentence	The I is engaged too strongly or too weakly	Presence
Astral body	Impulse to speech, word	Breathing disorders, all forms of breakdown in speech	Origin of illness (somatic illnesses), mood
Ether body	Alphabet, the sound	More specific speech disorders, for instance sigmatism	Disposition to illness, general state of health
Physical body	Production of the sound	Malformations, accidents	Symptoms of illness, diagnostic findings

On the basis of this diagram, the two principal fields of application for therapeutic speech and their relation to eurythmy therapy may be categorized.

First field	Second field
Speech formation for disturbances in the physical and functional levels of speech and the speech organs in the widest sense: articulation, voice, breathing disorders, and so on. More frequent in children	In this field, aetiologies lying in the astral body are treated; these often arise when the I does not take strong enough hold. Generally adults are more affected.
Therapy:	Therapy:
The healthy archetypes of the sound are applied. Feeling the speech instrument. By means of such feeling, the I takes hold of the archetypes of the sounds in the ether body. Thus, through the example of the therapist, disturbances in the patient's ether body and physical body are corrected. The essential principal is imitation.	On the one hand, the sphere of the spirit self works healing on the I, insofar as the latter is able to gain the upper hand in the astral body. On the other hand, the laws of the sounds, which are called up in the ether body, work from their side in a regulating way onto the astral body, and in a corrective way onto the physical body. The spirit self and the ether body work healingly when the I, from their regions, learns to call up the laws of the sounds.

In eurythmy therapy, the human being is placed directly into the pictorial laws of the ether body, which have been made accessible by the spiritual researcher. The starting point lies less in the astral body and the I than is the case with speech. The I places the body directly into these pictorial laws which have been adapted to the pathological process. A further basic difference is that speech is brought forth in the 'little human being' of the speech instrument, while with eurythmy it is the large human being of the limbs.

Numerous examples could be given for both the above fields, for both the therapeutic media and the course of therapy.

First field

An obese 13-year-old boy with Down's syndrome required treatment for his frequent wetting of himself during the day. The school doctor had found no organic reason, but had noticed that the boy breathed very shallowly. Because of this his breathing and awareness, along with his astral body, did not reach down as far as that region. Starting from this diagnosis in the first field (breathing), the sounds K and F were considered, as they allow the breath to be seated very deeply and have different effects. These consonants were supplemented by U, which of all the vowels works most strongly into the lower part of the human being. The syllables Ku and Fu arose, which were then developed into Kung-Fu, with strong contraction and releasing. These syllables, spoken dramatically, astonished the boy. They soon became fun to do and had the desired result.

In this case the breathing, and with it the insufficiently astrally-penetrated etheric body, was taken hold of from the level of the sounds. The I of the therapist was initially strongly challenged in trying to reach the child's inactive and moody astral body in a rigorous yet loving way, so that the latter could bring its own impulses to bear on the ether body. Through perception, this then brought about the desired control over the activity of the bladder.

Second field
In the case of a 50-year-old woman with ankylosing spondylitis and long-standing ulcerative colitis, no great change had been achieved through the direct levels of speech (first field). Working with the following texts was much more effective: episodes from the Heliand, the mediaeval religious epic; Goethe's poem 'Vermächtnis altpersischen Glaubens'; and texts by Albert Steffen and other modern poets. She learned many of these texts by heart. It made a deep impression when she described the help these poems were to her in the long and pain-filled period when she later underwent several operations for cancer. The strengthening effect of the spirit self on the I could be directly experienced here. In the case of somatic illnesses, both types of effect frequently appear at the same time, when in the same session exercises are followed by a text.

At the beginning we saw how the impulse to speech originates in the astral body, from where it takes hold of the other levels of speech. If it turns toward the I, that is where the consonants are formed, which 'arise between the I and the astral body'. If it turns toward the ether body it comes to the region where the vowels arise. In this sense speaking is nothing other than a continual interweaving by the soul of the regions of the I and ether body. It is the breath that is active, the messenger of the gods; it alone can create this union, in that it unites inner and outer worlds, above and below, the light of consciousness and the weaving of feeling.

Today, however, the astral body — the human soul — has 'lost' its feeling and will parts into the subconscious ether body, while thinking has inclined more strongly to the I, as described by Rudolf Steiner in the Speech and Drama course. The whole of the soul has been and is still the bearer of suffering. This makes it more understandable that so many causes of illness nowadays lie in the astral body. The breath, given wings by the content of the poem, becomes effective therapeutically. It unites thinking and the feeling will, consonant and vowel, and is thus the true Mercury, the healer.

The spirit self

In order now to consider the mysterious fifth level, that of the spirit self, we shall make another quotation our starting point.

> Were it left to the human beings themselves to hand on language to the next generation, man would pine away and perish. Being lives in language as truly as ever being lives in man himself. Along with speech and language something enters into man, wherein beings live whose whole life bears unmistakably the stamp of the spirit-self, even as in life man bears the stamp of the ego organization. These beings inspire us; they live in us through the fact that we speak.[4]

When the therapeutic aim is to strengthen the I (in practice a frequent indication from the doctor for speech formation), then the higher element mentioned in the quotation must be brought to bear: an element developed by the genius of language but not yet by human beings. The most diverse therapeutic experience shows that a particular poem, given and worked on in the situation of an illness, can be of great help to the I. The astral body, particularly in chronic illnesses, readily 'becomes accustomed' to being ill and thus becomes the trigger for ever more episodes of illness. This dynamic often lames the I. In such a situation, if the strengthened I can call up the astral body to a quite different and enjoyable activity, the pathological condition can be forgotten for the time being and in later phases can undergo a noticeable improvement.

Is it possible to grasp the region of the spirit self in a kind of diagnostic way?

This region comes to the fore when we observe a human being and see what their I has experienced and suffered through their destiny. Then we can approach with insight that sphere where speech has its origin.

In the poem, 'Song of the Spirit over the Waters' (Gesang der Geister über den Wassern) Goethe created a wonderful metaphor for how those spheres intervene. At the same time, the poem gives an insight into destiny and works as a therapeutic medium because it is inspired out of the region of the spirit self.

SONG OF THE SPIRIT OVER THE WATERS

The soul of man
Resembleth water:
From heaven it cometh,
To heaven it soareth.
And then again
To earth descendeth,
Changing ever.

Down from the lofty
Rocky wall
Streams the bright flood,
Then spreadeth gently
In cloudy billows
O'er the smooth rock,
And welcomed kindly,
Veiling, on roams it,
Soft murmuring,
Tow'rd the abyss.

Cliffs projecting
Oppose its progress —
Angrily foams it
Down to the bottom,
Step by step.

Now, in flat channel,
Through the meadowland steals it,
And in the polish'd lake
Each constellation
Joyously peepeth.

Wind is the loving
Wooer of waters;
Wind blends together
Billows all-foaming.
Spirit of man,

> Thou art like unto water!
> Fortune of man,
> Thou art like unto wind!⁵

Overcoming a hard blow from destiny is often the subject of good poetry. If, as a therapist, one understands something of the nature of this destiny, it can happen that one suddenly comes across just the right text and can accompany the seeking I of the other like a friend. Examples include alliteration from the Heliand, a hexameter, or something funny like 'The Hammer's Homecoming' from the Edda. Then the content and the poetry work together with the appropriate metre or style and can influence the other constituent parts of the human being in the way described above.

In his Fragments, Novalis indicates the therapeutic role of poetry.

> Poetry is the great art of constructing transcendental health. The poet is thus the transcendental physician ...
>
> It is completely understandable why everything becomes poetry in the end. Does not the world become soul in the end?

We may divine that our art, with the help of those geniuses of language, not only strengthens our I and transforms our soul. Its power also wills to pour itself into the outer world, contributing to its eventual transformation into poetry.

Some Experiences with Speech Formation

Ida Rüchardt

Every speech formation practitioner has their own way of teaching, their way of applying Rudolf Steiner's methods. Since speech formation is only in its early stages and deviations are possible, it would be important for all teachers to come together regularly in smaller or bigger groups (in Dornach as well as in Germany) in order to speak in detail about their teaching and their ideas, and also to remedy mistakes. Since this does not seem to be possible in the century of 'I have no time', I should like to put something down in writing out of my long experience.

I was given the sequence of the exercises during the beginning of my studies in Dornach in 1927. I have generally held to it, with exceptions when changes were called for with one or the other group of students. I have also composed exercises myself, when it seemed necessary for a student, or in order to introduce something that was lacking. This may seem disrespectful to Rudolf Steiner, but I have always taken his speech exercises, as well as his painting studies, as a foundation and as a stimulus to further composition. It struck me from the very beginning that there was a lack of vowel exercises. I am certain that Rudolf Steiner expected us to develop the exercises further.

I should like first to look at some details of the first exercises, for articulation. When one practises them with close attention over and again, there is a lot to say about them. The first exercise goes:

> Dass er dir log,
> uns darf es nicht loben[1]

How hard it is to begin an exercise with an impact sound and how liberating is the effect of the wave sound L in each line. One needs to concentrate on it. Then one concentrates on the vowels (which one goes through twice, with the exception of U). We may experience the whole world expressed by each vowel. And always our attention should be on the rhythm that is to be found in each exercise. Without rhythm there can be no speech formation. It is also very useful to do the exercise backwards, in two different ways.

> Log dir er dass,
> loben nicht es darf uns
>
> gol rid re ssad
> nebol tchin se frad snu

One could also rearrange the sentences. The second exercise:

> Nimm nicht Nonnen
> in nimmer müde Mühlen

An exercise for resonance and for the vowels I and U. M and N are nasal impact sounds and can easily be spoken too nasally; they should not get trapped in the head, as this can restrict the movement. They must be taken hold of lightly and moved with a lot of breath, otherwise they destroy the form of the speech. For I and U, one could also take:

> Prüfe dich Schüler
> übe mit Mühe

The third exercise is a proper sentence and indeed typical of German by virtue of the torn-apart verb:

> Rate mir mehrere Rätsel nur richtig

Then speak the whole exercise, treating the 'mehrere Rätsel' as a parenthesis, like a little loop in the big arc.

The fourth exercise is also important for the breath:

> Redlich ratsam
> Rüstet rühmlich
> Riesig rächend
> Ruhig rollend
> Reuige Rosse

One should be careful to carry the unaccented syllables along and breathe them through. It is also a wonderful exercise for R, but more of that later. As soon as the I becomes disengaged, the stream of breath is interrupted. One should also take care to use up all the breath in speaking the two words.

The fifth exercise is concerned with the fine difference between B and P, which are both lip sounds, yet differ in their dynamics.

> Protzig preist
> Bäder brünstig
> Polternd putzig
> Bieder bastelnd
> Puder patzend
> Bergig brüstend

For the sixth exercise, I use the L exercise in order to let the pupil experience the unfolding of the wave sound L, in the same way that it is so wonderfully expressed in the eurythmy exercise 'Hallelujah'.

> Lalle Lieder lieblich
> Lipplicher Laffe
> Lappiger lumpiger
> Laichiger Lurch

Then the first important breath exercise:

> Erfüllung geht
> Durch Hoffnung
> Geht durch Sehnen
> Durch Wollen
> Wollen weht
> Im Webenden
> Weht im Bebenden
> Webt bebend
> Webend bindend
> Im Finden
> Finden windend
> Kündend

I shall now quote from Creative Speech,[2] where Rudolf Steiner speaks about this exercise in contrast to the breath exercise, In den unermesslich weiten Räumen. It would be helpful to read the whole passage in the book.

Become aware of your breath by letting it go and following it through as it streams out. You need not be bound by any particular method. The method best suited to your organism will come.

Erfüllung geht ...

We have quite short lines here. Use up your breath completely in every line. Take a fresh breath before each new line ... Learn to become flexible with the help of the consonants and combinations of consonants ... Now you must become aware of the stream of your breath.

It is very useful to speak the words in reverse order, for example: Wollen – Nellow.

Unhindered by the sense one can draw out the inner qualities of the sounds to the full. Try to go with the oscillations of the double L to trace what it does with the O and the E. You have to learn from the sound itself what you must do in order to utter the sound. Try to hear with your whole being, to hear what the air does when you speak ...

What takes place in diaphragm, chest or head should take place unconsciously. You should not have the feeling at all of using the throat and other organs, but the air ...

You must learn from the sounds all there is to learn. The breath itself must be bought into play unconsciously when you sense the sound and, in sensing, hear.

Now we will do an exercise from which you can learn to understand what it means to enter into the tone and to make it live.

In den unermesslich weiten Räumen
In den endenlosen Zeiten
In der Menschenseele Tiefen
In der Weltenoffenbarung
Suche des grossen Rätsels Lösung.

Let the four lines gradually grow in intensity. To begin with, take your own tones with you so that everything sounds and reverberates together; then experience the air resounding outside you, into which you enter with the stream of your breath; learn to hear it; learn to know it as an entity into which you lay your own weak tone, which grows stronger through it and gradually becomes objective.

In the first four lines there lies an expectation which causes the tone to grow in intensity. It attains fulfilment in the fifth line, which expresses calm cognition emerging from will-filled consciousness.

> Let yourself fall!
> Erfüllung geht ...
> Now direct it!
> In den unermesslich weiten Räumen ...

You must acquire consciousness of your breath. You must acquire consciousness of how you hear the tone from within, not from without. Let it go, freed from intellect, then the sound falls into the stream of the breath and is carried along by it.

The essential consciousness of the sound, having been felt, is carried along as well. You yourself, being in it, hear from within and thereby fathom the tonal qualities in the word ...

The first exercise is well suited for finding yourself while letting yourself fall. There is a difference between a sudden plunge into the element of air, and the slow steering of a boat as in the second exercise.

To begin with, take the helm as an I-conscious being, then let yourself go, surrendering to the element that bears you. But feel your helm, the power of your I. It forms the barque that bears you, the barque of air, into which the stream of your breath is laid. Feel how it glides rhythmically along on the ripples and billows of the air. If you do this, you release something captive within you.

As a beginning exercise, Erfüllung geht is very difficult. For this reason, I have composed a preparatory exercise. The word Ach, at the beginning of a line, is an excellent way for the pupil who cannot yet speak on the breath at all, to venture out into the air. The exercise goes:

> Ach wie weit
> ja so weit
> O wie tief
> ja so tief
> Ho Gold
> so hold

Speak this really slowly on the breath outside yourself.

Yes, it is ho Gold; most speakers are not aware how important H is for formation. H, the breath itself, actually accompanies every sound. It is important to speak it in such a way that it takes hold of the vowel outside like a chisel, and is not squeezed out of the depths of the chest.

There follow some H exercises which I have made; it is good to practise them every so often.

A) Heller Habicht
hole heiter
heute hierher
Hunde Hühner
hinterwärts

B) Hundert Hunnen haben Hunger
Hundert Hunnen haben Hunger

C) Hände heben
hämisch hässlich
Hähne Hälse
Hering hält

D) Ach helft hellen Herzen
ach helft heftigen Herzen
ach helft heftigen hellen Herzen
ach helft heftigen hemmenden
hängenden hellen Herzen

E) Himmlisches Hifthorn
hilft Hyperion

F) Harrende Hasen halten am Abhang

Then Rudolf Steiner's exercises for speaking epic, paying attention to the forming of the H.

Halt! Hebe hurtig hohe Humpen!
Hole Heinrich hierher hohe Halme

Among the exercises for fluency there are combinations of sounds that only occur in the German language:

Pfiffig pfeifen pfäffische Pferde
Pflegend Pflüge pferchend Pfirsiche

Pfiffig pfeifen aus Näpfen
Pfäffische Pferde schlüpfend
Pflegend Pflüge hüpfend
Pferchend Pfirsiche knüpfend

>   Kopfpfiffig pfeifen aus Näpfen
>   Napfpfäffische Pferde schlüpfend
>   Wipfend pflegend Pflüge hüpfend
>   Tipfend pferchend Pfirsiche knüpfend

Many words in German which have Pf at the beginning, in the middle or at the end, have only a P in other languages.

>   Pfirsich – peach (English) – pêche (French)
>   Kopf – kop (Dutch)
>   Apfel – apple (English)
>   Pflug – plough (English) – plug (Russian)

In North Germany, the P is silent — they say, Ferd, Flaume.
An excellent exercise by Rudolf Steiner is the following:

>   Zuwider zwingen zwar
>   Zwei zweckige Zwacker zu wenig
>   Zwanzig Zwerge
>   Die sehnige Krebse
>   Sicher suchend schmausen
>   Dass schmatzende Schmachter
>   Schmiegsam schnellstens
>   Schnurrig schnalzen

The powerful Zw, the voiced S, and the Sh/Sch with M and N. Other than in German, the sound Zw appears only in Russian: zwet (colour); zwetok (flower); zwesti (to blossom). Instead of Zw, the English have Tw or Dw: twig (Zweig), dwarf (Zwerg), twenty (zwanzig).

An excellent fluency exercise for placement of the different impact sounds — palate, teeth, lips:

>   Ketzer petzten jetzt kläglich
>   Letztlich leicht skeptisch
>   Ketzerkrächzer petzten jetzt kläglich
>   Letztlich plötzlich leicht skeptisch

One should accompany it consciously with the breath. Other speech gymnastics exercises are (I will mention only a few):

>   Schlinge Schlange geschwinde
>   Gewundene Fundewecken weg

> Gewundene Fundewecken
> Geschwinde schlinge Schlange weg.

There one can learn the very important sound combinations Schl and Schw, as well as Ng, which can easily become enclosed in the nose.

> Marsch schmachtender
> Klappriger Racker
> Krackle plappernd linkisch
> Flink von vorne fort

> Krackle plappernd linkisch
> Flink von vorne fort
> Marsch schmachtender
> Klappriger Racker

Breathe out strongly with Marsch, then let the syllables run.

It is very useful to practise single words in order to be able to breathe through the sounds. One can begin with short words, like Erde, Asche, Ton.

The point here is to go through all the sounds consciously and to use up all the breath. Feeling should not be allowed to disturb by intruding. Then there is:

> Wasser Welle Woge
> Feuer Funke Flamme
> Luft Licht

Now come compound words, simple ones at first, then more complicated; they can be spoken in different ways. They can gain different nuances by the way one takes hold of the syllables more or less strongly.

> Waldesschweigen
> Wellenrauschen
> Windeswehen
> Sturmesbrausen

The German language has the possibility for such compound words; poets can always create more through their imagination.

Before doing vowel exercises, I like to do the exercise hum ham hem him, which I have expanded a little.

Hum ham hem him
lum lam lem lim
wum wam wem wim

Hung hang heng hing
lung lang leng ling
Wung wang weng wing

I have also added a few to Rudolf Steiner's vowel exercises.

Sturmwort rumort um Tor und Turm
Molchwurm bohrt durch Tor und Turm
Dumm tobt Wurmmolch durch Tor und Turm

This is also a good exercise for freeing the breath. One has to go through the vowels consciously, and on to the next consonant, while feeling everything that happens with the vowels on the way.

Grund und Ursprung
du schufst uns
du suchst uns um uns

Here one can sink right into the different nuances of the U.

Droben loht ein grosses Feuer,
noch verschont es das Gemäuer.
Hoch und rot und gross und voll
Sonnenross auf Wolken schwoll.

In Gottes Schoss
o Trost, so gross.
(From a poem by Christian Morgenstern)

O, wie fühl ich in Rom mich so froh. (Goethe)

Ö is very helpful, as its particular dynamic is to break through, something we need to strive for with all the sounds.

Höhnet die Spötter,
höret auf Götter,
löschet die Schöne,
lösende Söhne,

> krönet die Höhe,
> töne, o Böe.
>
> Öffne den umwölkten Blick (Goethe)

Then Ü.

> Lügen, trügen, hüben, drüben,
> schwülstge Blüten süss betrüben
> Kühle Lüfte mühend pflügen,
> grüne Früchte glühend rügen.

Then E and I have a different dynamic. Rudolf Steiner explains this by saying that E has something nervous about it when it is woven into other sounds. At the same time it is the sound that expresses fixed thoughts.

E is important for consolidating the speech organs, as it serves to send the nerve stream inward. With I, the power of the nerves immediately follows the stream of breath and works outward.

One needs to let this polarity work through the speech organization.

E appears in German particularly often — in this verse by Rudolf Steiner, for instance:

> OSTERN
>
> Steh' vor des Menschen Lebenspforte,
> Schau' an ihrer Stirne Weltenworte.
> Leb' in des Menschen Seeleninnern:
> Fühl in seinem Kreise Weltbeginnen.
> Denk' an des Menschen Erdenende:
> Find bei ihm die Geisteswende.
>
> Stand at the gateway to human life:
> see cosmic words clear written there.
> Live in the interior of the human soul:
> feel world beginning in its sphere.
> Think of the human being's earthly end:
> find in it the spirit's turning tide.[3]

It is hard to form E in the right way — it can easily be pressed so that it hinders the stream of breath.

Another exercise we have is a text by Julius Hey, recommended by Rudolf Steiner:

Schneebedeckte, feste Erde —
Lenzgeweckte erste Herde!
Ceres, Segenspendende —
Ew'ge, Verderbenwendende!
Sende den West dem Meer entgegen,
Spende der Erde schwellenden Segen,
Lechzender Herde quellenden Regen![4]

The following exercise, also by Hey and recommended by Rudolf Steiner, is useful:

Es streben der Seele Gebete
Den helfenden Engeln entgegen;
Entdeckend des Herzens Wehe,
Wenn Schmerzen es brennend verzehren!

The reader will know Rudolf Steiner's exercises for E and I:

Lebendige Wesen treten wesendes Leben

Wirklich findig wird Ich im irdischen Lebenswesen
Im irdischen Lebenswesen wird Ich wirklich findig.

Next there are some aids for speaking I:

Hier bin ich nicht,
im Ich ist Licht,
ich bin in mir,
wie blind sind wir,
für mich bin ich nicht,
für dich bin ich Licht.

A verse from one of Albert Steffen's poems:

Aber in der schwarzen Nische
seh ich Glimmerlichter stricheln,
immer wieder Silberfische
durch die Finsternisse sicheln.

I would just like to say that the vowel E is usually spoken particularly badly — it is pinched and not taken hold of by the stream of breath; the stream of speech is thereby impeded.

There is a very good but little known exercise for A and O. It frees the throat.

> Droben lag Rocca die Papa.
> Tonangebende Potentaten von hohem Range
> lobten Lage und Ort.
> Hervorragende Namen zogen manchen dort an.
> Auch Grafen Gonzaga und Goriola
> sassen droben an der Hoteltafel.
> Es folgten sodann Barone,
> solche von Adel und solche von Golde.
> Von Kolmar der Kommandant,
> ein Rotbart aus Colorado.
> Von Monaco Omar und Olga.
> Nora und Dora assen Orangen
> und tranken Mocca und Condorango.
> Ilona flocht Anemonen ins rote Haar,
> trollte lachend davon, um Korallen zu holen.
> Nora und Dora horchten auf der Goldamsel Sang.
> Horch Glockenklang und Choralgesang.
> Orkanartig tobten die Wogen bei Rocca di Sasso.
> Holla, da floh mancher vor Angst!
> Hallo, Holla?

Rudolf Steiner's A exercises particularly emphasize the long and short A; as does the well-known 'Barbara sass nah am Abhang,' also taken from Julius Hey.

Another helpful little exercise of mine:

> Der Berater im Theater
> ideal wie ein Aal.

Great care has to be taken with the diphthongs, which demand an even more differentiated movement than the vowels — Ei Au Eu Ai Äu. A diphthong may never be spoken as if it were turning back, self-contained, but as if it were dissolving into the air. As with everything artistic, it is difficult to describe — it must be heard and done.

I have added to Rudolf Steiner's exercises the end of a poem by Christian Morgenstern:

> dass dein volles Sein in mein,
> mein volles Sein in dein Sein Einlass fände,
> und so sich rein vereinte Sein mit Sein.

From a poem by Rilke:

> Ich aber will dich begreifen,
> wie dich die Erde begreift.
> In meinem Reifen,
> reift dein Reich.
> Ich will von dir keine Eitelkeit,
> die dich beweist.
> Ich weiss, dass die Zeit
> anders heisst als du.

From a poem by Goethe, for Au: Da staunen wir und traun dem Auge kaum.

For Eu (by me): Eure feuchte Eule leuchtet.

Another exercise I have composed: Blaue Weiten durchleuchten weise meinen Leib und Geist.

I would just like to mention here that the combination of the sounds B and L is very helpful. One should speak, Blaue Blume blüht in Bläue.

After the vowel exercises it is a good idea to speak the breath exercise considered earlier, In den unermesslich weiten Räumen.

In this article based on my personal experiences I cannot mention all the splendid exercises and remarks by Rudolf Steiner, which are in any case familiar to my colleagues, nor would I wish to. All I can contribute is what I myself have experienced, where this could be helpful. I should like to reemphasize this.

I found in Goethe's Achilleis an excellent extract for shaping the phrasing in sentences and subsidiary clauses:

> Gleich der beweglichen Schar Ameisen, deren Geschäfte tief
> im Wald der eilende Schritt des Jägers gestöret, ihren Haufen
> zerstreuend, wie lang er und sorglich getürmt war, schnell die
> gesellige Menge, zu tausend Scharen zerstoben, wimmelt sie
> hin und her, und einzelne Tausende wimmeln, jede das Nächste
> fassend und sich nach der Mitte bestrebend, hin nach dem alten
> Gebäude des labyrinthischen Kegels. – Also die Myrmidonen. Sie
> häuften Erde mit Erde, rings von aussen den Wall auftürmend. Also
> erwuchs er höher augenblicks, hinauf in beschriebenem Kreise.
> Like the mobile horde of ants, whose business deep in the forest
> the hurrying step of the hunter disturbs, destroying their heap, no
> matter that it took them long to build it with care, the convivial
> masses, scattered in a thousand hordes, swarm now hither and

yon, as scattered thousands are swarming, each one grasping their fellow and striving on for the centre, onward to the old building of their labyrinthine cone.

Thus the Myrmidons. They heaped up earth upon earth, piling up the wall in a ring from without. It grew thus straight away higher, up in the circle described.

For the placement exercises, I have found excellent examples in Schiller's Flüchtlinge, which should be spoken after Rudolf Steiner's exercises (Bei meiner Waffe, and so on):

LIPS:
In säuselnder Kühle
beginnen die Spiele
der jungen Natur.
Die Zephire kosen
und schmeicheln um Rosen,
und Düfte beströmen
die lachende Flur.

TEETH:
Wie silberfarb' flittern
die Wiesen, wie zittern
tausend Sonnen im perlenden Tau.

PALATE:
Wie hoch aus den Städten
die Rauchwolken dampfen.
Laut wiehern und schnauben
und knirschen und strampfen
die Rosse, die Farren,
die Wagen erknarren
ins ächzende Tal.

Those are the main placements, but there are many others which lie in between, which cannot be described, but must be done — spoken. One should never forget that speech lives in the etheric; could there ever be such diversity in the physical world? Different languages, dialects, the uniqueness of each speaker? Only when you know the sounds of many languages and their diversity are you able to approach the archetypal sound; this can be heard particularly in a chorus, where everything personal is swept away. It is difficult to experience in the German language, where the sounds are clear and barely susceptible of modulation; but magnificent when it does happen.

It is very important to practise proper, living speaking of prose, where particular attention must be paid to the treatment of subsidiary clauses, and to the structure, the 'values' as Marie Steiner said, in order to avoid the dullness of putting everything 'next to each other'. Schiller's prose is very good in this regard. I will quote a sentence:

> Jeder individuelle Mensch, kann man sagen, trägt, seiner Anlage
> und Bestimmung nach, einen reinen, idealischen Menschen
> in sich, mit dessen unveränderlicher Einheit, in allen seinen
> Abwechselungen, übereinzustimmen, die grosse Aufgabe seines
> Daseins ist.

> Every individual human being, one can say, bears within him,
> according to his disposition and destiny, a pure, ideal human being,
> the immutable entity of which it is the great task of his existence to
> be concordant with, in all the changes of life.

Fables are to be recommended; and Die Zeder by Goethe is very useful. Consciousness must stand behind everything, then the I can step in powerfully. A good exercise for the consciousness, put together from various sources is the following, based on the word Einst (once).

> PAST:
> EINST, da ich bittre Tränen vergoss ... (Novalis)
>
> Du wurdest EINST im Erdbeginn erhört ... (Steiner)
>
> Auch sie, die alten Gespielen
> wohnen wie EINST mir dir. (Hölderlin)
>
> PRESENT:
> Mir redet diese Flamme wunderbar.
> Von einer windbewegten Ampel Licht,
> Die EINST geglommen für ein nächtlich Paar,
> Ein greises und ein göttlich Angesicht. (C.F. Meyer)
>
> FUTURE:
> Erkennen wirst du EINST
> dich fühlte jetzt ein Gotteswesen ... (Steiner)

EINST zeigt deine Uhr das Ende der Zeit. (Novalis)

Jede Pein wird EINST ein Stachel der Wollust sein.
(Novalis)

EINST schauen meine Brüder auch wieder himmelwärts.
(Novalis)

If there are difficulties speaking the tongue R, I recommend the following exercises; beforehand, instead of speaking R, one speaks D.

d d d d d d d
Fort dort Kern gern Korn Dorn scharf darf

It is also very good to speak Redlich ratsam with a B before each word; also Rate mir mehrere Rätsel. Then:

d d d d
Brausende brummende brennende Braten

Die Fahrt bewahrt den Narren.
Den Wirt verwirrt das Klirren.
Dort kreisen die krummen Dornen.
Schreibe schreckliche Schritte.
Verschrobener schrulliger Schraben.

Die Narren verharren in Karren.
Die Bären verehren die Mähren.
Die Irren verwirren das Klirren.
Die Toren und Mohren rumoren.
Lemuren knurren und murren.

Trau treue Trine,
trau trüben Träumen nicht.
Treib trotzig triumphierend
fort das trübe Traumgesicht.
Trockne der Tränen
traurig trüben Lauf.
Trink trauten Traubensaftes
tröstend Tropfen drauf.

One could compose many more exercises, but usually a rolling R is achieved quite soon with these ones.

A sound which is nearly always spoken badly is W (V in English) — one hears either F or B. W is a blown sound which is related to the watery element. It is not for nothing that it starts words like Wasser (water), Welle (wave), Woge (billow). It needs the movement and dynamic of the English W, combined with the right German pronunciation. It is good to do the following English exercise:

>swan swam over the sea,
>swim, swan, swim,
>swan swam back again,
>well swum, swan.

The following exercises are also useful:

>Weben schweben beben
>wiegen schwiegen biegen
>Wahn Schwan Bahn
>Wein Schwein Bein
>and so on (develop fantasy!)
>
>Wellen schwellen bellen
>Wall Schwall Ball
>woll schwoll boll
>willen schwillen billen.

A pure S is something many people need, not just those who lisp. Rudolf Steiner gave the sequence N L D T, in which connection it is helpful to speak the following, one after another:

>Nimm nicht Nonnen ...
>Lalle Lieder lieblich ...
>Drückt die Dinge ...
>Tritt dort die Türe durch

Now some of my own compositions with a strong emphasis on the S:

>Liest Hans?
>Wacht Hans?
>Schlief Hans?
>Lacht Hans?

Wachs ist weiss,
Max beisst Lachs,
was das heisst.

Wie fass ich Wiesel?
Wo find ich Waffen?
Was schaff ich selbst?

The voiced S:

Ach sieh die singende See,
so sagte der sorgende Seemann,
Summend sanften Sang
und setzte sicher die Segel.

It has been my experience that people who have a weak, unclear S should practise F; therefore the following should be practised before beginning with the previous exercises:

Vom Vorigen fürchte nimmer
für findige Fünfheit
den feurigen Fund
Nimmer fürchte fünf fangende Finger
wenn findige fahrende Fante
vom Vorigen künden.

Fünf Finger fangen fähige Fische
Affen und Laffen die schaffen
Zu den Waffen rufen die Frommen
Feige faule Schufte raufen.

Further exercises for S Ch Sh/Sch Z:

Sie sitzt im Sessel und zischt
Sie singt süss und löst sich auf
Ach, lass das sein
Ich sass und ass.

Thinking of N L D T:

Hallt noch drinnen durch schaurige Nacht
lastende, sausende Hast?

Grollt nicht minder im Lande und harrt
deiner die wachsende Last?

Die Griechen suchen nach leuchtenden Edelsteinen,
doch die wachsen nicht auf Bäumen und Sträuchern.

I would advise strongly to concentrate on one word and how it appears in different contexts, requiring a completely different approach each time, even as far as the sounds are concerned.

One could take the word Herz (heart) as an example:

Schweig stille mein Herze (Be still, my heart. Mörike, Schön Rohtraut)
Herz in der Brust wird beengt (The heart in my breast is cramped. Hebbel, Nacht)
Sein Herz wuchs ihm so sehnsuchtsvoll (His heart swelled within him so yearningly. Goethe, Fischer)
Herz ich trinke dir Vergessen zu (Heart, I give you a toast to oblivion. C.F. Meyer, Lethe)
Sie tät' einen Schlag ihm auf sein Herz (She'd give him a blow on his heart. Herder, Erlkönigs Tochter)
Zum Opferdienst will ich das Herz mir rüsten / So wird dies Herz dir machtvoll Antwort geben (I'll gird my heart in readiness for the ritual / Thus will this heart render you mighty response. Steiner, Mystery Dramas)

The word Herz lives in a different sphere in each case; how intensely we experience it with Rudolf Steiner!

You will surely have noticed how differently one shapes something pictorial as compared to something audible. One should consciously practise the distinction. The following provide examples:

I see: A bright sunny day, a swaying field of corn
I hear: Hush, the somnolent flutes of death are sounding
I hear, I see: Listen, eight hooves are clattering up the mountain — two
    friendly riders!

In order to attain clarity about musical speaking, it is good to work on a text as both a song and a poem, for instance 'Ganymed' by Schubert and Goethe; or 'Frühling' by Wolf and Mörike. It becomes clear that musical tone relies on height and depth, which is not there in the case of the sound of speech, which only has movement and direction. When speaking musically one has to take care that it does not get stuck in the notes through constant movement.

It is important for every student to practise speaking for eurythmy during their training. This recitation gives them a foundation, but they must be corrected by an experienced teacher.

For experiencing the archetypal sounds, chorus speaking provides the proper training. In a well-trained chorus, the personal element disappears into the archetypal, so that one comes to a true experience of the sound.

One should always practise different rhythms! I cannot go into this here at any great length, but would just like to make a few suggestions. For the hexameter, which Rudolf Steiner particularly recommended, I suggest starting with Goethe distichs such as 'Weissagungen des Bakis' and 'Antechoir Form such nähernd'; also passages from the 'Roman Elegies'. One should study again and again what is said in Poetry and the Art of Speech about Greek and Germanic rhythms, and one should speak the examples. One should also practise recitation and declamation and experience these different worlds, which are often interwoven with each other, are extremely mobile, and may never be tied down schematically; even though there are many poems which belong clearly to one style or the other. There is always life and movement in art!

Speech formation gains a completely new aspect, as does rhythm, when one includes other languages. In fact, I would say that one only becomes fully aware of the unique character of the German language through the study of foreign idioms. The German language stands in a special position among the others. Most other languages have more or less differentiated sounds — vowels which adapt melodiously to the consonants and in doing so undergo considerable changes; consonants which attack the vowels or embrace them tenderly and, in these movements, go through surprising transformations. We can experience the influence of the landscape, the elements, the acuity of human reason. The beauty of other languages can appear here on a higher plane, refined by the power of consciousness.

Permit me to touch on the characteristics of some European languages, in order to go in greater depth into what I said about the German language. Who is not delighted by the melodious sound of Italian, when it is spoken beautifully? We meet a wealth of vocal modulations, guided by gently-spoken consonants, lifted here and there on a wave of double-consonants.

In French, on the other hand, we have gliding — one is reminded of the saying of Pierre-Charles Roy: 'Glissez, mortels, n'appuyez pas' (Glide, mortals, do not hold yourselves up) — glide into the polished and finished, into perfection. Here the vowels strive to change nuance, become diphthongs and enclosed in nasal sounds.

Polish is strongly formed. Hard and soft sibilants play with the turning nasal sounds. On the other hand, the Russian language flows calmly in indescribably melodious sounds — not for nothing does Russian have the same root for river and speech — reka and retsh. This language moves continually between two poles: the hard and the soft, between darkness and light.

In English we can experience an amazing diversity of vowels and differently-coloured consonants, which represents the elemental world with an inimitable power. The vowels, which fly, opening and closing, and even turn, are swooshed through by the consonants, themselves tempered by the watery element.

When we consider the German language, nothing of the sort confronts us. What do we find there; what is present? If we school our ear a little, the first thing that occurs to us is that German is the language of the centre. Here we have very clear vowels and diphthongs, and equally clear, hard, incisive consonants, accompanied by little modulation in the cadence, which gives foreigners the impression of a persistent staccato. But what a field of activity for the speech formation practitioner!

A new impulse as a shaper and former has to come in, which can only come out of human consciousness. Human beings themselves work at this language, mould it and awaken the beauty hidden within it. First they will turn to what lives between the sounds; they harken to the forces within which each sound lies embedded, and the awakening of these forces will be wonderful. Movement will go through the forces, which previously lay there next to each other, dead and isolated — first a movement within the sounds themselves, 'a sacred force and secret', and straight away relationships between the sounds will appear — this is how the miracle of enlivening through the human being takes place, through the liberated breath, guided by the I. The more boldly human beings engage themselves selflessly and unstintingly, the more colour, light and warmth will approach them, while ever wider perspectives open up. The beauty of the German language will become apparent. Not only in the sounds do we recognize its position; it also reveals itself in the sentence structure, which can only be taken hold of and carried by a wakeful I. Likewise in its capacity to combine words at will, as I have already mentioned. I should just like to add how it is particularly the very long words that can be formed in various different ways: wohlgesangdurchschwellt, allherzweiternd, Weltenseelengeister, according as one highlights this syllable or that.

In Rudolf Steiner's poetry there is an enormous number of such words. On the other hand a purely intellectual construction such as Lebensmittelkennzeichnungsverordnung (regulation of food labelling) is unbearable! Practising compound words increases inner mobility.

Goethe says (West-östlicher Divan):

> Das Wort erreicht, und schwänden Ton und Schall!
> Ist's nicht der Mantel neugesäter Sterne?
> Ist's nicht der Liebe hochverklärtes All?

> The word's attained, though sound and tone be gone!
> Is't not the mantle of the newborn stars?
> Is't not love's universe transfigured?

These lines encompass the whole world of the Logos, the whole realm of formed speech. It is not tone and clangour that can pierce through and reach their goal, be they never so full and loud — but the word, when it is sent forth on the freed breath through a human being's impulse, behind which stands an alert consciousness. Tone and clangour are overcome — the power does not lie in the physical — and an unbounded spiritual activity is revealed in the formed speech, and addresses the human being like a God-sent wakening call.

This formed speech is carried by a powerful movement and shaped into forms. Like the magnificent tracks of stars which follow higher laws, the most varied figures are inscribed into the ether — language becomes the 'garment of newly-sown stars,' of individual words, syllables and sounds, which emerge like shining stars from the great weaving of movement. As the stars float freely in the ether without support and are held in the life-stream of the spirit by their mutual relationships, speech resounds, borne by the I, without seeking support in the physical, but finding balance in the mutual relation of word, syllable and sound.

Now we come to the foundation of speech formation: taking hold, letting go, accompanying — which, when carried out in speech, give it a higher naturalness which ordinary, intellectual diction can never attain, because it expunges the sounds instead of allowing them to unfold. Does not the deepest and purest Christ impulse live in taking hold, letting go and accompanying? We are permitted to take hold of something, but only in order to let it go again, sheltered by our being; we let it go without turning our back on it, we accompany it as a selfless helper. Formed speech depends on this activity, which must never be separated from it, otherwise the 'love's universe transfigured' would be hurt. Speech, formed of the spirit, can do much to foster better relations between people as it is the archetypal art, as Rudolf Steiner pointed out. It arises in that the gods play on the human being's breath through the human heart.

As speakers, then, we live in our free breath in cosmic movement, in sacrificial love. Goethe coined this wonderful expression, anticipating the path of schooling given us by Rudolf Steiner and Marie Steiner for the spiritual progress of humanity.

If one is aware of all this, one may experience a deep responsibility as a speech formation practitioner. Something great is laid in our hands, and I would like to bring it to everyone's awareness through these remarks of Rudolf Steiner's:

> In the artistic forming of speech, the healthy working-together of body, soul and spirit is harmonized and revealed. The body shows whether it is able to incorporate the spirit in the right way; the soul reveals whether the spirit lives in it in a true way; and the spirit shows itself clearly in its direct physical effects. Those taking part in speech courses thereby experience anthroposophy as it is revealed — quite directly — through the activity of the human being. It could be seen as a test of anthroposophy that it has been in a position to enable the art of speech in its full significance to flourish once more, after being brought to a state of helplessness by the materialist view of life.[5]

Speech Formation in the Waldorf School

Ilse Schuckmann

What do you actually do? Is there enough work with speech formation to occupy one fully? Is there enough to do to justify a full-time position?

Such questions are often put to me. They show that many colleagues are not aware of the need for a speech formation teacher at a school. In order to awaken awareness for this and to encourage colleges of teachers to take up this issue, I would like to share something of my work in the Hanover Waldorf School.

Speech formation is a subject which needs to unfold quite freely in a school. It is not laid down in the timetable, at least not at the outset. In the course of their work, however, a speech formation teacher will naturally stick to the timetable they have made for themselves, like any other colleague. Nor is there a curriculum, such as exist for German, history or stories.

All this means that the work has to be shaped very individually, based on the needs of the particular school and on the capacities and gifts of the speech formation teacher. Some will concentrate mainly on class plays, others will work with individual children in a more therapeutic way, and yet others will work on speech with the other teachers. There is also recitation in the upper school. These areas cover the principal fields of work.

A passage from the Basle teachers' course (The Renewal of Education) has informed my work and led me to concentrate particularly on the second seven-year period:

> It is not just with the teeth that, out of our own nature as it were, we have once more to make something our own which we initially received through inheritance, it is also the case with something else; and that is, above all, with human speech.[1]
>
> The mystery of the development of human speech, as far as its essential nature is concerned, is really hidden from the modern

scientific mode of thought, in fact from the whole of modern science. It is not known that, just as the milk teeth arrive as a kind of inheritance from the parents, speech is acquired through a kind of external influence from the surroundings, via the principle of imitation, which then becomes an organic principle.

One learns to speak in the first years of life from one's surroundings. But the speech that is acquired in this way, and which is spoken by the child until the fourth, fifth or sixth year, has a similar relationship to the whole human being as the milk teeth have to the whole human being. Once someone has gone through puberty: what they actually have in their speech, what they speak, what becomes active in them in that they speak, is actually something that they make their own a second time ... What actually goes on continually in the whole human being in those important primary school years is a miracle — what goes on not just in the human body and not just in the human soul, but in the human soul body, in the soul of the body, year in, year out, month by month, in connection with making one's own inwardly what one has acquired in the way of speech externally from the surroundings in early childhood.

Whoever is able to observe in this field finds the following: in the first years of life up to the change of teeth one can see how the faculty of mental representation separates off, as it were, at the change of teeth, so that once the change of teeth is complete, conceptual ideation can then shape itself! While mental imaging withdraws at that time to a certain extent from the bodily nature and becomes an independent capacity of soul, what happens later, between the change of teeth and sexual maturity — although signs of it are apparent earlier — is that what we call the will withdraws from the whole organization of the child and becomes localized in the organization of the larynx and of speech. Just as the conceptual life presses inward and becomes an independent element of the soul life, in the same way the element of will becomes localized in what has developed from speech and its organs in the fourteenth or fifteenth year — with some children, of course, somewhat earlier.[1]

You can see from this that the second seven-year period is extremely important. The child lives in a process of continual creation and shaping of its individual speech; during this period one has the greatest opportunity to intervene helpfully. After puberty speech is already largely established so that it requires much greater activity by the young person if they wish to overcome their difficulties.

In the question-and-answer session 'On Speech Defects' in Creative Speech, Rudolf Steiner says:

> A real remedy for speech disturbances, for example, is to make proper use of the time between the seventh and fourteenth year, by gently bringing the sufferer to the kind of imitation I have described.

I work with children from Class 1 to Class 8 in such a way that I fetch them out of main lesson, as eurythmy therapists do, for fifteen to twenty minutes, individually or in groups. This happens three times a week for four to six weeks. The class teacher puts the children forward. They are either children with real speech disorders or those who need support or strengthening through speech. For instance, in the lower classes they would be children whose capacity for speech is quite weak. They can be helped relatively easily and often become more active and confident, also in their other lessons. Other children have speech that is too shallow and which easily becomes rigid and monotonous. Others again are very inarticulate or clumsy in their speech. When one has worked with them for a while, an improvement is most apparent in the way they recite their birthday verse before the rest of the class. Children whose speech has become unclear through long-term wearing of teeth braces are often in urgent need of help. Of course these difficulties cannot all be cleared up in four weeks. However, when one works with the children over and again in the course of their time at school, one can still give considerable help toward a healthy development.

This work, which can only ever benefit a few children, is supported to a great extent by working with colleagues. We prepare poems that the class teacher then does with the children in their class. It is good if the teacher has already prepared in Class 2 for speaking psalms in Class 3, or appropriate alliteration for Class 4 and hexameters for Class 5. Then a certain facility has already been acquired before the teacher begins work on this material with the class some months later. If someone has worked in speech on texts from ancient cultures or different historical periods, they will be able to speak about it from a different level of experience than if they have considered it only conceptually. The lessons, usually with two or three teachers during a school lesson, are not just confined to class teachers. Teachers from any field might be involved — kindergarten, arts and crafts, foreign languages, right up to upper school maths teachers. After all, the way a teacher speaks works right down into the developing organs of the child.

In the question-and-answer session mentioned above, Rudolf Steiner continues:

> You see, people speak to each other in ordinary life, but they notice very few ... of the imponderable effects passing from one person to another in speaking. But these effects are nonetheless there. We have become so abstract today that we actually only listen to one another in respect of intellectual content. Very few people have a feeling today for what it actually means when a person equipped with a rather more psychic-organic sensibility feels, when he has spoken with someone, how he continues to bear the other person's manner of speaking in his own speech organism to a high degree, consciously. Very few people today have a feeling for all that one experiences in this direction when one has to speak with four, five or six people one after the other, of whom the first coughs, the second is hoarse, the third yells, and the fourth is incomprehensible. For your organism follows all that as well. It goes on vibrating in sympathy, it experiences all that, too.

During the time when they are acquiring speech themselves, children are much more susceptible to what is described here in connection with adults.

Then there is also helping with class plays — I mainly concentrate on Class 8.

In the upper school, work with individual pupils continues on the basis that those with speech difficulties arrange with the main lesson teacher when they will go to speech formation. It is entirely voluntary, and some pupils carry on into the final year.

Help with recitation in main lesson in the upper school is at the request of the teacher, if they do not wish to do it themselves. Working with the pupils on texts which particularly lend themselves to being recited can be a real help, for instance, in the Faust block in Class 12.

This report is intended to show one way in which speech formation can be integrated into the life of a school and what its tasks are. As I said at the beginning, this will happen differently in different schools. It is my concern that over time more and more colleagues feel the need for a speech formation teacher, and that there will be enough people who wish to unite themselves with this task and prepare themselves for it. Only in this way will it be possible to counter the horrifying disappearance of the power of speech among children. The objection that some schools do not have the means for such a post is unrealistic in my view. If the need for nurturing speech is recognized it will also prove possible to realize it.

No school, for instance, would think of abolishing eurythmy because it could not be afforded. Admittedly Hanover is a large school, with parallel classes from Class 1 to Class 13, six kindergarten groups and a training course for Waldorf kindergarten teachers who have speech formation twice a week. There is so much to do here in the realm of speech that it can hardly be covered by one person alone. At a school without parallel classes, a speech formation teacher would have a field of work which they could just about manage.

4

Reports on the Development of Therapeutic Speech since 1976

Report on the Further Training Course for Speech Formation Practitioners

Caroline Wispler

Following a conversation between physicians and speech formation practitioners in February 1976 that called for a more consistent and co-ordinated approach to therapeutic speech, the initiative was taken to hold a further training course at the Goetheanum. This course took place in October/November 1976.

In this three-week course, Dora Gutbrod and Ingeborg Mau took a first step toward fostering a broader and clearer awareness of the therapeutic task of speech formation, within the context of the School of Spiritual Science at the Goetheanum. Individual speech formation practitioners had been working for a long time with doctors in schools, special needs schools, clinics and therapy centres; they had gathered a wealth of experience and knowledge which they shared here. For colleagues already working therapeutically, mutual concerns could be shared and knowledge increased; for colleagues new to this field of work it served as orientation. It also formed the foundation of a course of training in therapeutic speech.

Through the contributions of the many physicians taking part, participants gained an insight into the overwhelming variety and scope of the human, cosmic and esoteric aspects of speech.

It is not possible to reproduce the wealth of content and, above all, the practical advice and descriptions of actual cases that contributed to the variety and colourfulness of the conference. Insofar as it is possible for an individual participant, I shall try to focus on a few aspects of the whole conference which show how its anthroposophical basis and methodological approach might point the way to a further training course for speech formation practitioners, which needs further development.

Each day began with practical speech formation exercises with Dora

Gutbrod. We worked on Rudolf Steiner's speech exercises in such a way that we always tried to experience and manifest the spiritual presence of the sound, syllable, word and sentence movements. We schooled our ears to perceive ever more closely the difference between articulating and intoning the sounds — the formed breath resonating and moving together with the external, objective power of the sounds. We worked intensively at the inversion of the activity that was about to happen: from where one is striving to articulate speech from within and breathe it outward; to something higher, which lies in the in-breathing, immediately before speech. We sought to unite ourselves spiritually with the sequence of sound pictures that was to be spoken, and their meaning, so that they can take hold of the stream of breath and manifest within it. When it works, there is a feeling of effortlessness, as if it has happened independently of our own effort. When we are unsuccessful, we realize more and more clearly how the speech-will is 'taken over' by the concept, which has converted what should only happen through the movement of the sounds into a fixed image. Meaningful and powerful bodily movement can wrest the formative will away from that and liberate it into the movements of the sounds.

As far as content was concerned, we worked on the basic kinds of movement in earth, water, air and fire, using verses and mantrams from the Rudolf Steiner's fourth mystery play, also Goethe's poems on clouds and each day a poem by Rudolf Steiner about the nature of speech. Dora Gutbrod brought alive for the participants Marie Steiner's mighty endeavours, which contributed to the atmosphere and to our work together. All of this formed an experiential backdrop to the lectures and conversations, which helped deepen our understanding. All who took part were very grateful to Dora Gutbrod for consciously putting speech formation's artistic path of schooling in the foreground of our practical work of renewal. Continually following this path is the first condition for any work seeking to unfold the healing power of speech.

Alongside the artistic path of experience, taking up speech formation as a therapy based on anthroposophy calls on us to comprehend the human being as a speaking being. The necessary scientific approach, as Dr Paul von der Heide explained, lies not so much in the communicable results as in the path to them; in the age of Michael, this path can be followed anew by each of us. Taking up this question in a real way, which involves the human being, the world and history in equal measure, is only possible through a schooling of the consciousness, the starting point of which Rudolf Steiner describes at the beginning of The World of the Senses and the World of the Spirit. Starting from this inner foundation, the image of the human being in relation to speech unfolded from ever different perspectives.

The basis for many of the lectures was the idea that the speaking human being shapes the stream of breath in such a way that the play of the sounds in space can unfold in the out-breath, guided by the I of the speaker, which makes use of its corporeality, the organs of speech, as an instrument. Speech enables what is spoken to free itself from the speaker in such a way that it takes on an independent existence in space, which the listener can dip into and understand. Nowadays speech is heard and spoken, but mostly so utterly at the service of human information that it requires a great deal of attention even to notice its independent existence in relation to the human being. A first step toward this is to become aware that speech, although it is very much the direct revelation of an individual human being, could neither have come about through that human being alone, nor have developed from self-consciousness. (This was the starting point for Dr Frits Wilmar's lecture.) Speech is a being that is independent of the human being, even though it serves humans. People can encounter it through speaking and listening and become acquainted with it. However one needs to have the will to free oneself from the content that is being communicated and to immerse oneself in its ways of moving, its gestures, colourings, melodies, rhythms, sound-pictures and so on; and to discover the forces of the vowels and consonants as the principles of the world of speech. This means awakening more deeply to the still relatively young, undeveloped sense of the word; this awakening can occur in the encounter with the being of speech, as Dr Georg von Arnim showed in his lecture.

In linguistics, on which speech and language therapy is based, this awakening is prevented by the misplaced theory that speech is a system of signals for the purposes of communication, based on social convention. The physiological, psychological and sociological processes of hearing, comprehension and speech may still be susceptible of research, but not the objective forces of speech, which are revealed through the study of anthroposophy to be the 'creating, forming and shaping universal word,' and which have placed the human being in the whole nexus of the world and its process of development, where they wish to elevate the human being to be a co-creator as Dr von Arnim and Dr von der Heide showed.

Dr Albert Gessler described how the stream of the out-breath involves a creative, generative process, which reaches right into material substance. In the out-breath, all the components which form protein, which is the substance of everything living, are present, albeit in different proportions, combined with warmth: carbon, oxygen, nitrogen and hydrogen. This breath, exhaled from within, is still virtually alive for a brief moment. As a physio-etheric stream it offers the forces of the sounds a fleeting opportunity to incarnate in a living, manifest form. Nitrogen plays a crucial role in this process; it is the only substance which is exhaled untransformed, in the same state as when it was inhaled into the lung. All the other substances combine with the blood and are transformed within the human being. Nitrogen is a substance of the utmost elasticity and cosmic mobility, the basis of the pure, macrocosmic astrality, which, in the human being, Lucifer and Ahriman have been unable to separate from its origin, and which does not unite itself with the human being's individualized astrality. The spiritual forces of the vowels and consonants are at work in it, described by Rudolf Steiner as the creative forces of the planets and the zodiac.

All speech which maintains the connection to the formative forces of the starry astrality, even where the sound is fettered, has an objectivity beyond the individual's personally astral formative process; our speech can be more whole and sound than we ourselves are. At this point, speech formation's approach to therapy became clear: the breath is able creatively to bring about the connection with the starry astrality, which itself can correct and heal the individual astral body, which is what makes us ill (Dr Gessler, Dr von der Heide).

The more freely the breath and the more openly the personal will to speak strive forth beyond themselves and release themselves, the more purely the macrocosmic forces of the sounds can incarnate and appear in the sense world in a fleeting 'dance'. Their presence works back on the speaker; Rudolf Steiner calls this process 'physiologizing back'. What arises as an independent sound formation becomes a being through the vowel substance and consonant formation. This being, which is like a second, 'fully sentient human being' (as Rudolf Steiner described it), separates out from the human being and works back on it, renewing it, like a true archetype of its misaligned being. It thus becomes clear that, particularly also when working therapeutically with speech, one must strive to become free in the air, to be released into the movements of speech themselves and venture 'beyond one's fingertips'; otherwise the renewal from the starry astrality cannot be fulfilled. There is an aspect here whereby a difference in approach becomes clear compared to eurythmy therapy, where what is set free in artistic eurythmy is taken back and turned back on the organism. How is the human being able to create this new being of speech?

Dr Wilmar described how the human body, particularly the organs connected with speech and the breath, are built up before birth through the forces of the planetary spheres and the realm of the zodiac, of cosmic vowel and cosmic consonant. Cosmic music and the cosmic word, resounding, form the physical and etheric bodies, remaining present within their structures, though having fallen silent. The ether body, which is an individualized copy of the structure of the whole cosmic ether, and thereby of the world word, is impressed, like a seal, into the physical nerve and sense system, so that the physical brain appears as a crystallized image of the world word. Every time the human being speaks, speech appears as a process of bringing out the dormant power of the sounds concealed in the ether body; it is part of the birth of the etheric human being in the air and on the stream of the breath. The air appears as the element in which the outer starry forces of the sounds, working creatively in the present, meet again their past deeds, now become image. For with every in-breath the air unites, through the mediating oscillation of the cerebrospinal fluid (the theme of Dr Gisbert Husemann's lecture), with the individual, crystallized imagination of the world word which is at rest in the brain.

In the lecture, 'The Investigation and Formulation of the World Word in In-breathing and Out-breathing,' Rudolf Steiner describes each breath as a 'sensing of light by tone.'[1] The speaking of language itself takes place in the arena of and in collaboration with the earthly human being.

However this process, which should make the human being the servant of the word and at the same time its co-creator, has become subject to the capriciousness of the purely earthly purposes of the human being, and awareness of what lies behind it has been lost. Human speech has lost its free creative power: on one hand it is fettered to the physical speech organs; on the other, what lived in it as the bringing-forth of names — whereby the human being was united with the essence of things in an artistic, cognitive process — was banished almost completely to the superficial objectivity of the sense world, becoming the means to an end within a world that is accessible through technology. In this connection, Dr Wilmar described how this situation is the fruit of a deed whereby Ahriman intervened in human development during the Atlantean period and, with the help of the whole movement organization, concentrated human speech, which was originally far more spiritual, into the specialized processes of the functioning of the larynx and of audible speaking.[2] Knowing that the way we speak is a gift of Ahriman's, which today is becoming one of the ways in which he fetters the human being to what is earthly, might awaken a sense of the responsibility connected with all forming of speech; this is the motivation for a way of speaking which consciously wishes to wrest itself away from this rigidifying grasp to take its place at the beginning of a cultural therapy and cultural renewal.

I will now outline the different approaches that were shared in the work we did on aspects of curative education, Waldorf education and social therapy.

In curative education there is the task of helping children with special needs on their way into incarnation through bringing on and giving an impulse to their speech. When learning to walk, the child makes its whole movement organization its own; learning to speak involves a new stage of taking hold of oneself. An almost painful contraction into the larynx takes place, which represents the utmost concentration of the whole movement organization. Dr Hellmut Klimm spoke about how the force with which speech engages, frees itself from the grip of this contraction and creates a new relation to the world, to other human beings and to one's own incarnation. This step is only possible on the foundation provided by the sense of the word. Only those who can perceive speech and recognize it as such, who can listen, can speak (the theme of Dr von Arnim's lecture). It is very important for the therapeutic speech practitioner to discover whether a child has undertaken this preparatory process of awakening which underlies all speech: being able to perceive the sounds of speech for what they are; it can happen that a child is even able to imitate consonants and vowels in a babbling sort of way, without being able to grasp what they express. Movement is the way to this. The sense of the word is a metamorphosis of the sense of movement. Where a capacity has arisen through the mediation of a sense and has then withdrawn from consciousness, a potential for higher perception opens up: perception of speech arises out of the capacity for movement (Ursula Ostermai).

Dr Rudolf Braumiller also mentioned this connection when he explained the interrelation of finger games, gesture, gait and a person's whole way of moving, and their reflection in the way they speak. One methodological aspect of speech work is to cultivate movement and spatial orientation exercises, both as preparation and to accompany speech. It is not possible to repeat all the suggestions and practical examples here. However, it is important to notice, even in this preparatory stage, where there might be disorders that would interfere with the learning of speech. The astral body might be so sucked into the activity of movement that there is no space left for anything higher; or it can be completely absorbed in nervous and sensory processes, leaving it unable to take hold of the movement organism; or it might be that the echo-like accompanying oscillation of the larynx when listening to speech does not happen. For this latter, children should also watch eurythmy, so that the oscillation may be stimulated by looking at the outer movement (Ursula Herberg).

It is also possible that a child may be unable to tolerate the process of becoming awake to and concentrating on speech; or that the fine fluid currents in which the forces and qualities of the sounds oscillate etherically are impaired (Dr von Arnim). The other approach to fostering the activation of speech proceeds through an enlivening of the senses toward a loving uniting of oneself with the world. This becomes particularly clear with children who, while they have the bodily preconditions for speech, appear to be so 'engaged' in their soul life that they are unable to open up to the world. In the interplay between release in a well-regulated capacity for movement and a trusting union with the world of the senses, speech begins to be released on the stream of the breath, which is the actual healer which unites both poles. It cannot be influenced directly through practice; breathing is learnt through the feelings. It must be enlivened by the things and processes of the world. The teacher's breathing, guided always by feeling, accompanies the child and can enliven their breathing through imitation. Ursula Herberg spoke about Steiner's descriptions of certain forces of the lip, teeth, tongue and palate sounds have releasing or consolidating effects on various speech disorders, whereby the image of a karmic difficulty becomes apparent.[3]

The main themes running through the reports from work in schools were: guiding the children into the formative forces of speech; the step from speaking correctly to speaking beautifully, and to an experience of the power of speech in the three parts of the second seven-year period. In connection with the structure of the main lesson blocks in the curriculum, work with speech can help open up and enliven the content given by Rudolf Steiner as an answer to the inner questions living in the children at that age (Ilse Schuckmann). It is also important to use speech with certain speech and general behavioural disorders. Gertrud Maliga reported on her work using different rhythms with children with a lisp or a stammer — 'compassion that has become organic' or 'anxiety that has become organic'; she also worked with the lyrical, dramatic and epic styles in speech. Christa Slezak's presentation showed that the inner aim for work with children between the ages of seven and fourteen is to lead them into the life of speech in such a way that they do not lose their connection with the genius of language in later life. Today this connection is more and more under threat, and with it the relation to the spirit of the age (according to Dr von Arnim). Only on this basis will it be possible to overcome certain speech disorders.

A second challenge is presented through the lives of children in large cities with all their technology, where their natural sense perception has largely been destroyed. Particularly because speech stands so close to the perceptible world, it can help to re-enliven this world once more. It can once again become the instrument which reestablishes contact between human beings, which is becoming ever more endangered. Speech is the being which lives between human beings, mediating, setting boundaries, and uniting on a higher plane. The collaboration between Christa Slezak and Dr Braumiller, a school doctor, showed how one can proceed from the perception of an individual pupil and an understanding of the peculiarities of their constitution, character, temperament and speech to targeted provision of therapeutic speech. They described a whole array of individual children including diagnosis and therapy. This was complemented by a lecture by Dr Hanno Matthiolius which showed the incarnation process of the child, from the embryonic period through to the early seven-year periods, through a study of rhythms of the pulse, diaphragm and chest breathing. Their eventual harmonizing in a rhythm of 4:1 only comes about as a result of complex development processes. This was illustrated by means of many graphs.

Ingeborg Mau described how work with adults does not involve the application of speech's formative forces in line with the developmental laws of the seven-year periods, but rather the finding of the individual's own language. By taking hold of its own language, the I can learn to work into the structure of the component parts of its human being — harmonizing, regulating, maintaining their coherence — in order to be able to live within them. Through its forms, speech is able to mediate the regulating laws of thinking, feeling and the will from without. Through an experience of the sounds, by filling a gesture with feeling, and by elevating ideas into images, it can also enliven interest in what the senses mediate, thereby bringing liberation from confinement in one's own being. The canon of Rudolf Steiner's exercises as an organism, which portrays in speech the totality of the human being, is the basis of the work, as well as the whole realm of poetry. In poetry human beings, in that they strive beyond themselves, are united with the forces of the future coming from beyond death. Through speech there is a great potential here for catching up on experience of the world, from which the human being can be cut off by illness, or for reactivating it through memory. In later life there comes a fundamental transformation in human development, and this is important for the relationship to speech. It is liberated more and more from what is purely individual and can unite itself with the spirituality of language itself, on the basis of the metamorphosed ether and physical bodies. It is possible to work on anthroposophical texts which, through their content, take hold of and apprehend the ways of the I.

The examples given from the work with patients showed clearly how individualized the course of treatment with speech needs to be when adults are involved; although here there are still laws at work, albeit less obviously. Dr Rudolf Treichler described in some detail the inner course of the seven-year periods in human life and revealed the origins of potential crises.[4]

The accounts of Simone Gétaz and Ina Krediet made a deep impression on the whole conference. Their very personal descriptions of their experiences and diverse approaches to their human encounter with ill children and adults gave the listeners a feeling for the role of destiny in these encounters, which were guided by the higher being of speech, encompassing both therapist and patient.

The following methodological approaches and suggestions for future work were put forward in the contributions and conversation: therapy means recreating and experiencing the patient so strongly within oneself that healing forces are summoned up which then become manifest. It is a high ideal, which can only be aspired to through rigorous schooling. Real forces are at work which want to be drawn in and consciously recognized in each individual case. What is actually being called on is the power of intuition in the anthroposophical sense of the word. In his education lectures Rudolf Steiner described how, through studying the human being from the point of view of spiritual science, the right idea would come to mind when one was in the classroom. Researching and wrestling for conceptual clarity about the nature of the human being and the world, then forgetting its content and taking it into sleep, transforms inner forces and makes them receptive to effective, helpful intuitions in the midst of everyday practical problems. One aspect of further training, therefore, would be the anthroposophical study of the human being, as has already been begun in this course from different points of view. One could look at how the gesture of a sound can be recognized in the structure of different organs. Dr Friedrich Lorenz broadened this to a 'science of the world', in which the forces of particular sounds were described in relation to human organs, earthly elements, the ethers, zodiacal forces and the workings of the hierarchies. It would be particularly important to think in terms of an anthroposophical physiology of speech, for which Dr Husemann's lecture on the connection of the organs of speech and breathing with the movement of the cerebrospinal fluid, for instance, paved the way.

A further subject for study is the oft-repeated remark that Rudolf Steiner's speech exercises are, as an entity, the whole human being in the realm of speech. Beginning with a description of the movements of the sounds in the goitre exercise, An Angegebenes sieh innig hin, and of the rhythmical structure of the exercise, Sahst du das Blass an Wang und Mund, Ingeborg Mau showed how one can begin to find one's way in this area. All the other studies of the elements of speech should also be included here. Dr Günter Schönemann encouraged the study of rhythm, initial rhyme and terminal rhyme in connection with rhythms and temperaments in the human being, with reference to the book Rhythmen der Sprache by Martin Georg Martens.

The counterpart of schooling through study is schooling through observation. The necessity of training one's ear for the variety of what can be perceived in speech in education and therapy was emphasized again and again by doctor and therapeutic speech practitioner alike. How is a person's speech: loud, soft, high-pitched, deep, sluggish, dull, sparkling, musical, staccato, tinny, flowing and so on? How is their speech connected with their being, their way of moving, their impulses of will, their line of thought, the flow of their feelings? To what extent is it physiologically compacted and mineralized? Does the vowel or the consonant element predominate? Do certain qualities of the sounds predominate? Is a person's 'sound mood', as mentioned in the Speech and Drama Course, audibly perceptible?

It is clear that these tasks have their foundation and focal point in a continual practice of speech; only thus is it possible to get to know ever more deeply the power of the sounds and the way they work. They themselves must become our teacher. The beginning of therapeutic work is where our own speech can find the way toward 'etherization'.

At the end of the three weeks, the participants found that the almost overwhelming multiplicity of ideas had coalesced into a coherent whole, and every detail nevertheless pointed to new tasks. This has been confirmed by the new impulses that have since arisen, and by a gradual assimilation of what has come out of the conference. Deepest gratitude to all who brought the conference about is combined with hope for future work in the spirit of what was begun here.

The Further Training Course has been held almost every year from then. Since 2001 artistic speech formation was included as the therapeutic speech conference was the only one being held for speech formation practitioners.

The Origins and New Beginning of Therapeutic Speech

URSULA OSTERMAI

The therapeutic application of speech formation has a long history. Some of Rudolf Steiner's first speech exercises from before the 1920s have targeted indications and a clearly described effect. Targeted application with patients began under Ita Wegman through the work of Martha Hemsoth, whose activity is highlighted at the beginning of this book.

Until 1976, certain individuals practised therapeutic speech in the strict sense of the word: Ina Krediet, Simone Gétaz, Gertrud Maliga, Ilse Schuckmann, Ingeborg Mau, Christa Slezak-Schindler, Ursula Herberg and Dora Gutbrod. They worked independently of each other, but with a doctor, and really laid the foundation in their different fields of application.

Ursula Herberg worked intensively in curative education. Her work with therapeutic speech is documented in a book first published in 1978.

Then there was the pedagogical speech work done by Christa Slezak-Schindler at the Kräherwald School in Stuttgart, by Gertrud Maliga at the Waldorf School in Reutlingen, and by Ilse Schuckmann at the two Waldorf schools in Hanover. Ingeborg Mau worked for over thirty years at the Friedrich Husemann Clinic in Buchenbach. Their work really set the standard for those of us who began later.

They were all individuals who took their idealism, enthusiasm and will to work with speech formation out into the cities and their institutions, some following their own impulse, some Marie Steiner's.

Dora Gutbrod, who worked at the Goetheanum, also had a great deal of initiative. After she had retired from stage work, she discussed with her close friend Dr Madeleine van Deventer her wish to develop therapeutic speech formation out of artistic speech formation. She treated many patients in the Ita Wegman Clinic and achieved miraculous results, without perhaps really knowing why. As a further initiative she gathered colleagues and invited doctors to a small conference at the Goetheanum in 1974, with about sixty speech formation practitioners and physicians. I was twenty-nine then, and overwhelmed by the mood of euphoria which prevailed. There were passionate as well as sceptical exchanges of ideas, but everything was carried along on a tide of enthusiasm for this new departure. (Our conference in 1976, by contrast, was more sober and businesslike.)

A small preparatory group formed to organize the conference, of which Dora Gutbrod, Ingeborg Mau, Ursula Herberg, Ilse Schuckmann, Barbara Stelling and I were members. We were joined later by Helen Heberer, Christiane Starke and Dietrich von Bonin, and by many of the colleagues who still attend the conferences today.

Distinguished physicians gave us further training (one could almost say that they actually trained us). At any event, that is how it seemed to me. Why does a child not speak? Dr von Arnim answered this frequent question by guiding us into the relationship between movement, sense perception, understanding and destiny in the child concerned.

Dr Gisbert Husemann presented the metamorphoses of the forms of the larynx in a wonderful way. We hung on his every word, fascinated; he was a born actor!

Dr Rudolf Treichler introduced us to work with psychiatric patients, along with Ingeborg Mau — the etheric organization of the organs in relation to psychopathological soul states. A series of physicians from the Friedrich Husemann Clinic presented clinical pictures. I could mention much else. We were given a wealth of studies of the human being and of medicine, which was always put in relation to the speaking human being.

Other physicians, too, like Gotthard Starke, Frits Wilmar, Paul von der Heide, Madeleine van Deventer, Friedrich Lorenz and Albert Gessler, among others, took part in this continual further training. Their personal interest in speech formation, and the fact that they practised speech themselves, made it all directly relevant. Conference reports came about, as well as articles on the different tasks of speech formation practitioners in schools, special education and social therapy, and as independent practitioners.

In 1976, Dora Gutbrod offered a supplementary training in speech therapy for trained speech formation practitioners, but there was little response. The speech formation training at that time concentrated solely on drama. Interest in speech therapy, however, began to increase perceptibly, occasioned by the variety of the tasks which awaited young speech practitioners in the social field. In 1979, developments at the Goetheanum brought about a definite concentration on drama at the Speech Formation School there. This induced Dora Gutbrod to offer a basic training in speech formation, with a further training in therapeutic speech, under the auspices of the School. In 1978, Christa Slezak-Schindler had also started a training in therapeutic speech. The following year, Alanus College offered an additional foundation year for therapeutic speech as a fifth year of study.

The whole situation of training opened up and expanded within a short time. When Dora Gutbrod died in 1989, and after my ten years of collaboration in her training, I founded the Dora Gutbrod School for the Art of Speech which continued until 2009.

Where are we now?

A review can only be fruitful if it leads to a preview of future prospects. What has changed compared to the early days? What have we achieved up till now? What are the tasks and challenges that confront us?

Back then, thirty years ago, the dawn of therapeutic speech came out of deep and fundamental artistic experiences on the part of speech formation practitioners and out of a certain artistic maturity. We wanted to make available to others what we had experienced as a blessing. There was an overabundance in the artistic, whereas therapeutic awareness was just beginning.

Today the wealth of experience that has been gained has led to understanding, recognition and research. Medical knowledge, social-therapeutic competencies and the results of scientific research have been attained and are now available. We know the therapeutic moment and the therapeutic process; we read case histories and make diagnoses; we work with or without a physician and we document the treatment. Health insurance is involved; professional associations have been formed; and professional profiles have been drafted. We have achieved much, although there is still much to do. After all, thirty years is just a beginning for a new movement. It is like breathing, which is a pendulum-swing: we breathe out into the world; then we must breathe in again so that the phrase 'art therapy' can remain a reality.

Eighty years ago speech formation as an art was born entirely out of anthroposophy. It was still warmed through from the presence of Rudolf Steiner and Marie Steiner. All the artists still lived off the great experiences they had gained.

Today the echoes of that time have finally died away. We have to create everything from within ourselves and represent speech formation and therapeutic speech solely out of our own individuality. In the past, questions like the following did not arise. Is it actually possible without anthroposophy? What is anthroposophic art? Is anthroposophy one spiritual stream among many, and do not all roads lead to Rome? Am I aware of my source? Today it is up to us to answer them.

In the past the art of speech was going through a problematic development. Audiences found it weird. Pupils at Waldorf schools dreaded this art form: this drawn-out, measured singing and quavering, in a kind of speech-song. Speech formation had lost its good name.

Today there is still rejection. Speech formation as an artistic activity is increasingly vanishing from schools, seminars and conferences. We have to deal with people who condemn speech formation because it does not appeal to them, who think it ghastly, without ever having tried it for themselves. Only their own experience, however, can convert them. We have the task nowadays of persuading people verbally, as we cannot compel teachers, physicians and others to try it for themselves. Without this, however, nothing will happen. In the early days, the physicians all did speech formation themselves, which fired their enthusiasm and was the impulse for their personal commitment to therapeutic speech.

Compared with the early days, we face different problems: politics and the health service; a dramatic acceleration in the pace of cultural decline; and an extensive dulling of consciousness through television, computers and other media. We are confronted by loss of speech and its downfall, which gives us completely new tasks.

The questions asked during the conversation in February 1976 between physicians and speech formation practitioners like 'Could a therapeutic speech training be combined with a eurythmy therapy seminar?' or 'What does the path to a focused training look like?' have been answered. Paths of training have been created. At the Dora Gutbrod School, the basic medical content of the training was given to eurythmy therapy students and therapeutic speech students jointly.

We still have some intensive work in front of us to find answers to the two questions posed by Dr van Deventer: 'How can physicians participate in the experiences of speech formation practitioners?' and 'What is the standing of therapeutic speech practitioners in circles beyond anthroposophy?'

The earlier magnificent artistic achievements of the pioneer speech formation practitioners, from which the drama work arose, will come to life again in future in the personal experiences of speech gained by individuals. Speech gives self-awareness; it awakens the process of self-healing; it strengthens the will for life and the capacity to shape it — insofar as the practitioners of speech formation or of therapeutic speech do not lose sight of art; know that they are working in art; and never cease to continue learning artistically!

Thus we stand today at a new beginning, different to that of eighty years ago: one that can become a renewal of the original beginning.

Notes

Introduction
1 Barbara Denjean-von Stryk and Dietrich von Bonin, Anthroposophical Therapeutic Speech, Edinburgh 2005.
2 Oral communication by Susanne von Bonin to the Editor.

Martha Hemsoth
1 Dr Madeleine Petronella van Deventer, June 23, 1899 – Jan 23, 1983. Close colleague of Ita Wegman, subsequently Medical Director of the Clinical Therapeutical Institute (later called Ita Wegman Clinic).
2 Correspondence between Martha Hemsoth and Ita Wegman is reprinted by kind agreement of the Ita Wegman Archive. Correspondence between Martha Hemsoth and Marie Steiner is reprinted by kind agreement of the Executors of Rudolf Steiner's Estate, Dornach.
3 Emmichoven, Who Was Ita Wegman? Vol. 2.
4 Gracia Grace Ricardo (March 14, 1871 – Sep 28, 1955) was a singer and singing teacher. Through a pupil, she met Rudolf Steiner and anthroposophy, and was a friend of Matthilde Scholl for many years. She founded the Arlesheim Laboratories in America to make Weleda medicines more widely available. It is conceivable that this passage in the letter refers to this project, as Martha Hemsoth's husband, Wilhelm, had trained in business.
5 Mien Viehoff (Jan 8, 1895 – Nov 28, 1973). Born in Amsterdam, trained in Zurich and Holland in arts and crafts and bookbinding. She later studied singing and the violin. Close friend and colleague of Ita Wegman. Until the latter's death she worked at the Clinical Therapeutical Institute in Arlesheim, mainly in administration.
6 Dr van Deventer's report on Martha Hemsoth was kindly made available by Emanuel Zeylmans van Emmichoven.
7 Siegfried Pickert (June 3, 1898 – March 12, 2002) was one of the three founders of anthroposophic curative education. He studied German, History, Philosophy and Education in Posen (now Poznan), Jena and Berlin, and took part in the Christmas Conference of 1923 and the Course for Young Doctors. Rudolf Steiner gave the Curative Education Course following a request from Franz Löffler, Siegfried Pickert and Albrecht Strohschein. On Steiner's advice, Pickert took the examination qualifying him to teach in middle schools. With financial support from friends, Ita Wegman enabled the acquisition of Hamborn Castle; Pickert moved in in 1931 with forty people with special needs and a few co-workers.
8 Esoteric work on the mantrams given by Rudolf Steiner for the First Class of the School of Spiritual Science.
9 Emmichoven, Who Was Ita Wegman? Vol. 2.
10 Emmichoven, Who Was Ita Wegman? Vol. 3.
11 Typewritten page, kindly made available by Edith Guskowski.
12 The essay was given by Dr van Deventer to Emanuel Zeylmans van Emmichoven on

February 20, 1982.

Hildegard Jordi
The brief autobiography and the essay on therapeutic methods were given by Hilde Jordi to her friend Helene Pflugshaupt of Berne.
1 Steiner, Speech and Drama, lecture of Sep 13, 1924.
2 This text is attributed to Rudolf Steiner; different versions are in circulation.
3 Translated by Peter Patterson

A Therapeutic Exercise: An Angegebenes sieh innig hin
1 Archive number A5633, reprinted by kind agreement of the Executors of Rudolf Steiner's Estate, Dornach.
2 Rudolf Steiner, From Comets to Cocaine, lecture of Dec 2, 1922.

A Second Therapeutic Exercise: Richtig recht rechnen
1 First published in Degenaar, Krankheitsfälle.
2 Oral communication by Christiane Starke.
3 Roche Lexikon Medizin, Urban und Fischer, 2003.
4 Steiner and Wegman, Extending Practical Medicine, Ch. 19, eighth case.
5 Denjean-von Stryk and Bonin, Anthroposophical Therapeutic Speech, pp.81f.
6 Steiner and Wegman, Extending Practical Medicine, Ch. 19, eighth case.
7 See the chapter, 'The Fourfold and Fivefold Nature of the Human Being,' p. 139.

A Third Therapeutic Exercise: Ich atme Kraft des Lebens
This chapter was first published in Das Goetheanum, April 19, 1970.
1 Willi Kux (Feb 6, 1902 – March 26, 1976). Eurythmy teacher. From 1932 entrepreneur in Dortmund and co-founder of the Centre for Social Pedagogy there.
2 Steiner, Mantrische Sprüche, Seelenübungen 2, p.128.
3 Steiner, The Being of Man and his Future Evolution, lecture of Nov 10, 1908.

Reminiscences of Rudolf Steiner
This chapter was first published in Das Goetheanum, April 19, 1970.

Esoteric lesson
This chapter reproduced from Steiner, Esoteric Lessons 1904–1909, (translated by James H. Hindes) pp. 243ff, by kind permission of SteinerBooks, USA.

Upright Walking, Speech Movement, Eurythmy
First published in Das Goetheanum, Feb 27, March 6 and 13, 1977.
1 Stein, Zur Kultur der Seele.
2 Steiner, Das Ewige in der Menschenseele, lecture of April 15, 1918, p. 268
3 See also Heinrich von Kleist, On the Marionette Theatre, an Essay.
4 Steiner, Speech and Drama, lecture of Sep 6, 1924.
5 Steiner, The Redemption of Thinking, lecture of May 24, 1920.
6 Steiner, Eurythmy as Visible Speech, address of Feb 16, 1920.

The Fourfold and Fivefold Nature of the Human Being
This chapter was originally given as a lecture at the Congress on Research Methodology in

Therapeutic Speech Formation, March 12–15, 1998, Herdecke, Germany.
1 Steiner, Speech and Drama, lecture of Sep 5, 1924.
2 Steiner, Eurythmy as Visible Speech, lecture of June 25, 1924.
3 Steiner, Speech and Drama, lecture of Sep 15, 1924.
4 Steiner, Education for Special Needs, lecture of July 4, 1924.
5 Translated by A.S. Kline.

Some Experiences with Speech Formation
Written in Summer 1971
1 These and all subsequent exercises by Rudolf Steiner from Creative Speech.
2 'Speech exercises with explanation,' in Steiner, Creative Speech.
3 Steiner, Breathing the Spirit. The translation is by Matthew Barton.
4 Reusch and Hey, Der kleine Hey.
5 Steiner, Die Konstitution der Allgemeinen Anthroposophischen Gesellschaft, report of Aug 3, 1924.

Speech Formation in the Waldorf School
1 Steiner, The Renewal of Education, lecture of April 20, 1920.

Report on the Further Training Course
1 Steiner, The Sun Mystery, lecture of April 1, 1922.
2 See Steiner's lecture of September 2, 1916 in The Riddle of Humanity.
3 See Steiner, Speech and Drama Course, lecture of Sep 22, 1924.
4 Treichler lectures were written up and published (in German) Das Goetheanum (Nov 21, 28, and Dec 5, 1976).

Origins and New Beginning of Therapeutic Speech
1 König, et al. Sprachverständnis und Sprachbehandlung.

Bibliography

Bonin, Dietrich von see Denjean-von Stryk, Barbara, and Dietrich von Bonin
Degenaar, A.G., Krankheitsfälle besprochen mit Dr Rudolf Steiner [Medical case studies discussed with Rudolf Steiner] Klinisch-Therapeutisches Institut, Stuttgart, Germany 1939.
Denjean-von Stryk, Barbara, and Dietrich von Bonin, Anthroposophical Therapeutic Speech, Edinburgh 2005.
Emmichoven, Emanuel Zeylmans van, Who Was Ita Wegman? A Documentation, Mercury Press, USA.
Hey, Julius, see Reusch, Fritz.
König, Karl, Georg von Arnim, and Ursula Herberg, Sprachverständnis und Sprachbehandlung, Freies Geistesleben, Stuttgart 1986.
Lorenz-Poschmann, Agathe, Die Sprachwerkzeuge und ihre Laute, Dornach 1983.
—, Therapie durch Sprachgestaltung, Dornach 1981.
Martens, Martin Georg, Rhythmen der Sprache, Verlag am Goetheanum, Switzerland 1997.
Novalis, Fragmente und Studien, Reclam, Germany 1984.
Reusch, Fritz and Julius Hey, Der kleine Hey: Die Kunst des Sprechens, Schott Musikverlag, Mainz 1997.
Roche Lexikon Medizin, Urban und Fischer, 2003.
Slezak-Schindler, Christa, Künstlerisches Sprechen im Schulalter: Grundlegendes für Lehrer und Erzieher, Bund der Freien Waldorfschulen, Stuttgart 2007.
Stein, Heinrich von, Zur Kultur der Seele: Gesammelte Aufsätze, Cotta, Stuttgart 1906.
Steiner, Rudolf. Volume Nos refer to the Collected Works (CW), or to the German Gesamtausgabe (GA)
—, The Being of Man and his Future Evolution (CW 107) Rudolf Steiner Press, UK 1981.
—, Breathing the Spirit, Sophia Books, Forest Row, 2002.
—, Die Konstitution der Allgemeinen Anthroposophischen Gesellschaft und der Freien Hochschule für Geisteswissenschaft (GA 260a) Dornach, 1987.
—, Creative Speech (CW 280) Rudolf Steiner Press, UK 1978.
—, Education for Special Needs, The Curative Education Course (CW 317) Rudolf Steiner Press, UK 1998.
—, Esoteric Lessons (CW 266/1) 1904–1909, SteinerBooks, USA 2007.
—, Eurythmy as Visible Speech (CW 279) Anastasi, Weobley, UK 2005.
—, Das Ewige in der Menschenseele: Unsterblichkeit und Freiheit (GA 67) Steiner Verlag, Dornach 1992.
—, From Comets to Cocaine (CW 348) Rudolf Steiner Press, UK 2000.
—, The Healing Process: Spirit, Nature and our Bodies (CW 319) SteinerBooks, USA 2010.
—, Health and Illness (CW 348) Vol. 1, Anthroposophic Press, USA 1981.
—, Human Values in Education (CW 310) SteinerBooks, USA 2005
—, Introducing Anthroposophical Medicine (CW 312) Anthroposophic Press, USA 1999.
—, Karmic Relationships, Vol. 8 (CW 240) Rudolf Steiner Press, UK.
—, Mantrische Sprüche, Seelenübungen 2 (GA 268) Dornach 1999.
—, The Redemption of Thinking (CW 74) Anthroposophic Press, USA 1983.

—, The Renewal of Education (CW 301) Anthroposophic Press, USA 2001.
—, The Riddle of Humanity (CW 170) Rudolf Steiner Press, UK 1990.
—, Speech and Drama (CW 282) SteinerBooks, USA 2007.
—, The Sun Mystery and the Mystery of Death and Resurrection (CW 211) SteinerBooks, USA 2006.
—, The World of the Senses and the World of the Spirit, Rudolf Steiner Publishing Company, UK 1947.
—, and Ita Wegman, Extending Practical Medicine, Fundamental Principles Based on the Science of the Spirit (CW 27) Rudolf Steiner Press, UK 1996.
Stryk, Barbara Denjean-von, see Denjean-von Stryk, Barbara and Dietrich von Bonin

Index

ankylosing spondylitis 147
apical catarrh 99, 110
Arnim, Georg von 185, 188f, 194
asthma 107

back muscles 124–26
back-pain 64–71
Baumann, Elisabeth 74
Baumann, Paul 74
bedwetting, wetting 146f
bipolar affect disorder 51–59
Bittlston, Adam 27
Bonin, Dietrich von 99, 105, 139, 194
Braumiller, Rudolf 190
Braun, Adam 73
Burckhard, Willy 38
Bürger, Gottfried August 56

chorus speaking 171

Degenaar, Dr A.G. 99
Demosthenes 33f
Denjean-van Stryk, Barbara 13, 89, 105
depression 42–50
Deventer, Madeleine Petronella van 12, 17, 21f, 24f, 27, 73, 193f, 196, 199
Dionysius of Halicarnassus 34

Edda 150
Emmichoven, Emanuel Zeylmans van 11
English language 157, 171
eurythmy 132f
Eymann, Prof Friedrich 39

French language 171f
Froböse, Edwin 39, 76, 113

German language 156, 158, 165, 170f
Gessler, Albert 185f, 194
Gétaz, Simone 191, 193
Glöckler, Michaela 11
Goethe, Johann Wolfgang von 123, 136, 144, 149, 163
goitre 101
Grund, Erna 78
Gutbrod, Dora 12f, 73–85, 183f, 193–95

Gutbrod, Rolf 73f

Hahn, Herbert 142
Hebbel, Friedrich 49, 57, 81–83
Heberer, Helen 194
Heide, Paul von der 184–86, 194
Heliand 150
Hemsoth, Martha 11, 16, 17–29, 30, 33
Hendewerk, Kurt 12, 39f, 78, 85
Herberg, Ursula 188f, 193f
Hey, Julius 160f
Husemann, Gisbert 12, 123, 187, 194
hyperventilation 107

Jordi, Hilde 11f, 37–40, 41

Klimm, Hellmut 188
Kolisko, Eugen 27
Krediet, Ina 191, 193
Kugelmann, Margarete 21
Kugler, Walter 13
Kühn family 75
Kux, Ralph 109
Kux, Willi 105, 108, 109

larynx 127–32
Lorenz, Friedrich 191, 194
Lorenz-Poschmann, Agathe 11, 102

Maliga, Gertrud 189, 193
Martens, Martin Georg 192
Marwitz, Gerhardt 84
Matthiolius, Hanno 190
Mau, Ingeborg 183, 190f, 193f
Metaxa, George 111
Molt, Emil 73f
Morgenstern, Christian 79, 162
mother tongue 141f, 144

Novalis (Friedrich von Hardenburg) 150
Nunhofer, Dr Karl 26

Ostermai, Ursula 13, 73, 188, 193f

Pals, Lea van der 39
Pflugshaupt, Helene 12

Pickert, Siegfried 22, 199
Polish language 172
Pörksen, Gunhild 13

Ranzenberger, Hermann 89
Redlich, Bevan 78
Redlich, Gerdtrud 39
Ricardo, Garcia 19, 199
Rilke, Rainer Maria 162
Roy, Pierre-Charles 171
Rüchardt, Ida 13, 151
Russian language 157, 171

Sabunde, Raymond de 134
Schiller, Friedrich 164f
schizophrenia 59–64
Schönemann, Günter 191
Schubert, Karl 74
Schuckmann, Ilse 13f, 175, 189, 193f
Schuurman, Max 77
Schwebsch, Erich 74
Selg, Peter 13
Slezak-Schindler, Christa 11, 189f, 193, 195
speech defects 177
Sponholz, Günther 21, 26, 73, 83
Starke, Christiane 99, 194
Starke, Gotthard 194
Steffen, Albert 84, 161
Stein, Heinrich von 123
Stein, Walter Johannes 74

Steiner, Marie 12, 17–21, 27, 29, 39, 75–85, 109–11, 113, 165, 173, 184
Steiner, Rudolf 12, 18, 74f, 95, 101, 105, 109–12, 115, 123, 135, 153, 160, 173
Stelling, Barbara 194
Stockmeyer, Karl 74
Stryk, Barbara Denjean-van see Denjean-van Stryk, Barbara
Stuten, Jan 78, 109

Thomas Aquinas 133f, 136
Thylmann, Victor 17
thyroid gland 90–95, 101
Treichler, Rudolf 74, 190, 194

Unterbusch, Ralf 13, 89, 99

Viehoff, Mien 18f, 199
Vreede, Elisabeth 23, 27

Walser, Peter 41
Wegman, Ita 16, 19–29
Wilmar, Frits 185–87, 194
Wispler, Caroline 13, 183

Zeylmans van Emmichoven, Emanuel see Emmichoven, Emanuel Zeylmans van

Anthroposophical Therapeutic Speech

Barbara Denjean-von Stryk and Dietrich von Bonin

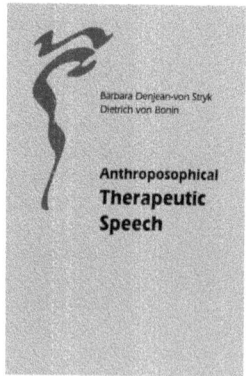

Written for speech therapists and physicians, this book gives a precise, practical summary of anthroposophical therapeutic speech.

Speech formation, or creative speech, is based on the ancient art of recitation and drama, and was revived and fundamentally redeveloped by Rudolf and Marie Steiner in the early 1920s.

The therapeutic work is based on speech exercises and indications on how to use them, which were given by Rudolf Steiner.

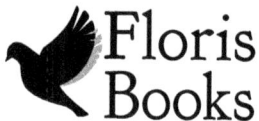

For news on all our **latest books,** and to receive **exclusive discounts, join** our mailing list at:

florisbooks.co.uk/signup

Plus subscribers get a FREE book with every online order!

We will never pass your details to anyone else.